SUPERVISOR
Training Manual for Healthcare Security Personnel

Third Edition

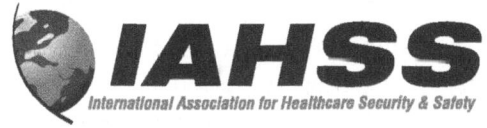

International Association for Healthcare Security and Safety

A program of the Council on Education of the IAHSS

Editor in Chief
Evelyn Meserve, CHPA

Editor
Nancy B. Williams, MS

Supervisor Training Manual for Healthcare Security Personnel, Third Edition

International Association for Healthcare Security and Safety (IAHSS)

© 2007, 2004, 1997 by the International Association for Healthcare Security and Safety
All rights reserved. First edition 1997, second edition 2004, third edition 2007
Reviewed 2012

Printed in the United States of America

Warning: The *Supervisor Training Manual for Healthcare Security Personnel* is fully protected under the copyright laws of the United States of America. All rights, including videotape, motion or still photographs, audio recording, and rights of translation into foreign languages, are strictly reserved. Nor may any part of this material be produced or used in any form or by any means, electronic or mechanical, including photocopying, printing, or otherwise recording, or by any informational storage and retrieval system without written permission from the Association. All inquiries or knowledge of violations regarding these rights should be addressed to the Association:

International Association for Healthcare Security and Safety
Post Office Box 5038
Glendale Heights IL 60139
Telephone: 630/529-3913 (888/353-0990)
Fax: 630/529-4139

Contributors of chapter material contained in this book are listed at the beginning of each chapter and in the consolidated contributor list. The consolidated list identifies current and former contributors, in alphabetical order. They are all persons knowledgeable in healthcare security operations and management. The material presented, and the validity of such material, is the sole responsibility of the contributors. Questions or comments concerning the material should be directed to the Council on Education of the IAHSS. All such comments or questions will be forwarded, by the Council, to the contributor for review and action as may be deemed appropriate.

Students are advised that any cost involved for instruction above and beyond this publication that the student deems necessary to prepare for the certification examination will be the sole responsibility of the student.

The Supervisor Training certification program offered by the IAHSS is presented for general educational purposes. Completion of this program is intended to signify cognition of course material by the participant. Program completion is not intended to imply any form of licensure or to warrant performance of any individual certified under the program. The IAHSS assumes no liability for the performance of any individual certified under the program.

Contributors

The IAHSS is pleased to acknowledge these security professionals for their contributions to the *Supervisor Training Manual for Healthcare Security Personnel*, Third Edition.

Tracy L. Buchman, MS, CHSP, CHPA
Hospital Safety Officer/Safety/Risk Management
University of Wisconsin Hospitals and Clinics
Madison, Wisconsin

Scott Buff
Training and Investigations Division
Carolinas Healthcare System
Charlotte, North Carolina

Alan J. Butler, CHPA
Director of Security
University of Wisconsin Hospital and Clinics
Madison, Wisconsin

John Driscoll, CHPA, CPP
Assistant Director, Police and Security
Massachusetts General Hospital
Boston, Massachusetts

Stuart G. "Fletch" Fletcher, CHPA, CPP, MBA
Corporate Director of Public Safety
Catholic Healthcare West (CHW)
Pasadena, California

Stephen W. Gaunt, MBA, CHPA
Director, Safety, Security, and Parking
Hoboken University Medical Center
Hoboken, New Jersey

Jon Hallaway, CHPA
Operations Manager
Harris County Hospital District
Houston, Texas

Anjanette Hebert, CHPA
Director, Security, Safety and Emergency Preparedness
Lafayette General Medical Center
Lafayette, Louisiana

Russell Jones, PhD, CHPA, CPP
Director, Protective Services
Albert Einstein Healthcare Network
Philadelphia, Pennsylvania

Chris Leibfried, CHPA
Director of Security
North Shore University Hospital
Manhasset, New York

Paul Mains, CPP
Director of Security
Florida Hospital
Orlando, Florida

Evelyn Meserve, CHPA
Director, Safety and Security Services
CaroMont Health/Gaston Memorial Hospital
Gastonia, North Carolina

Bonnie S. Michelman, CPP, CHPA
Director, Police and Security
Massachusetts General Hospital
Boston, Massachusetts

Dennis Parr, CHPA, CPP
Vice President
Hospital Shared Services
Denver, Colorado

Thomas A. Smith, CHPA, CPP
Director, Police and Transportation
University of North Carolina Health Care System
Chapel Hill, North Carolina

Bryan Warren, CHPA
Manager, Training and Investigations Division
Carolinas Healthcare System
Charlotte, North Carolina

Robert "Mickey" Watson, CHPA
Manager, Security
Sarasota Memorial Health Care System
Sarasota, Florida

Tony W. York, MBA, MS, CHPA, CPP
Senior Vice President
Hospital Shared Services
Denver, Colorado

The IAHSS is also pleased to acknowledge those who contributed material to the second edition of this manual. The current edition builds on information developed for that edition. The organizational affiliations noted here indicate contributors' status at the time of their contribution or, if known, their current status.

George Breshears
Security Safety Manager
Portneuf Medical Center
Pocatello, Idaho

John Connelly
President
Longwood Security Services, Inc.
Brookline, Massachusetts

James Costello, CHPA, CPP
Director, Security Safety
St. Francis Hospital
Roslyn, New York

Charles Dowell, CHPA
Security Manager
Calvert Memorial Hospital
Prince Frederick, Maryland

Jeff Karpovich, CHPA, CPP
Security Director
Carolinas Medical Center
Charlotte, North Carolina

Anthony McClure
Safety Manager
Presbyterian Hospital of Dallas
Dallas, Texas

Constance Packard, CHPA
Associate Director, General Services
Boston University Medical Center
Boston, Massachusetts

Anthony Potter, CHPA-F
Director, Security
Forsyth Medical Center
Winston-Salem, North Carolina

Nick Radu, CHPA
Director, Security and Police
Henry Ford Health System
Detroit, Michigan

Lynne Smith
Healthcare Security Services
Denver, Colorado

Paul Steiner, CHPA, CPP
Director, Security/Parking
Akron General Medical Center
Akron, Ohio

The International Association for Healthcare Security and Safety

Editorial and Book Publishing Team
IAHSS Staff:

Jim Balija, CAE	Executive Director
Nancy Felesena	Executive Assistant

Editors

Evelyn Meserve, CHPA	Editor in Chief
Nancy B. Williams, MS	Editor

Production Staff
Stenson Bauer Communications, Inc:

Mary Beach	Project Manager
Doug Taylor	Production Manager
Jennifer Reddy	Proofreader

How to Use This Book and Apply for Certification

The International Association for Healthcare Security and Safety (IAHSS) has the basic purpose of promoting professionalism in healthcare security and safety. Founded in 1968, this not-for-profit organization has members throughout the United States and other countries.

The Council on Education is responsible for the Association's training programs. Basic Training certification for security officers is a fundamental part of the training program. The *Supervisor Training Manual for Healthcare Security Personnel* is the third part of the Association's Progressive Certification program. This manual prepares individuals to complete the requirements for Supervisor Training certification. The manual is an edited collection of manuscripts (chapters) prepared by directors and supervisors of healthcare security or other persons considered to be highly competent in their field.

The Commission on Certification is responsible for the Association's certification programs. The Commission develops, monitors, and maintains the certification examinations for the IAHSS.

Using the Manual

The manual is divided into chapters. Each chapter contains the following:

- Learning objectives
- Text material
- Bibliography
- Study questions

The manual may be used for group or individual instruction. An instructor may use the manual in a classroom learning environment. Students in a study group can work through the manual. A student can also use the manual to study independently.

Self-directed Learning

Self-directed learning requires strict self-discipline. We encourage you to be diligent in your studies. In this way, you will achieve the maximum return for your time and effort.

When using the manual in self-directed learning, proceed at your own pace in the following manner:

1. Thoroughly read the individual chapter
2. Reread the chapter, underlining the important information relative to the objectives stated at the beginning of the chapter
3. Complete the review questions at the end of the chapter
4. Verify your answer by finding it in the chapter

Obtaining Certification

When you complete training based on this manual, you may apply to the IAHSS for Supervisor Training certification. The certification exam is a monitored, closed-book test consisting of 50 multiple-choice questions. The test can be taken on paper and mailed in or taken electronically, in which case you receive instant results.

To take the test, you must submit a completed "Application for Supervisor Training Certification Examination." Applications for the online and mail-in test are included at the back of this manual. You can also obtain applications and more information at www.iahss.org.

Re-certification

Once you have been certified, you must be re-certified within five years. You may apply for the same level of certification. Visit www.iahss.org for details.

Your Comments

The Council on Education of the IAHSS solicits your comments, suggestions, and questions concerning this manual. The Commission on Certification solicits your comments, suggestions, and questions concerning the Supervisor Training certification process. Contact the IAHSS and give us your thoughts.

Preface

Welcome to the third edition of the *Supervisor Training Manual for Healthcare Security Personnel.* The IAHSS is proud to provide this educational resource for today's professionals. An easy-to-use and up-to-date study guide, the manual helps prepare safety and security personnel to address the special needs of healthcare institutions. This resource helps prepare security personnel to take the IAHSS Supervisor Training certification examination.

In this edition, you will find much new material and many worthwhile changes. The Council on Education, regional and chapter leaders, and interested members have provided valuable input to guide our work on this revision. The new edition addresses several areas that members expressed interest in seeing in the manual. Again with this edition, we have drawn on experienced professionals in the field of healthcare security operations and management as authors and reviewers.

Changes with This Edition

Those of you familiar with the previous edition, please note that the manual has been updated and expanded to reflect the changes in our profession. The new edition is worth reading cover to cover.

New Chapters. Chapters discussing new issues that healthcare security personnel are apt to be affected by have been added. New topics are covered in their own chapters:

- Crime prevention programs
- Training plans and programs
- Security operations
- Emergency procedures
- Supervisor development

Expanded Material. Many chapters also provide more detail than in the previous edition.

Stronger Presentation. Throughout the book, we have focused on making the text easier to read and study. The editors have emphasized the use of plain language and made the organization of ideas as clear and direct as possible. To promote learning, we changed the look of the text and called out main ideas, key concepts, and subtopics. Information is now easier to find when you are looking for something specific. The questions at the end of the chapters now reflect examples of the certification exam questions.

The Value of Certification

The *Supervisor Training* manual is one component of the IAHSS Progressive Certification program. Through this publication, the IAHSS has endeavored to present the body of knowledge appropriate for those working in today's fast-paced, ever-changing environment. Studying this material develops your ability to grasp the essentials of security and safety in the healthcare environment.

Healthcare security supervisors must ensure their officers are competent to provide for the safety and security of all persons in the healthcare facility. Making sure the officers provide the best protection possible—for those who work there, those who receive care there, those who accompany or visit patients, and those whose work brings them on site—is the security supervisor's responsibility. Security supervisors have a second responsibility: to ensure that security officers know how to protect property. The security supervisor's role is to ensure his or her officers are comfortable and willing to do the job needed. The material in this manual provides needed information to the supervisor to accomplish those responsibilities.

Today's Professionals. Healthcare security personnel face challenges both old and new. The IAHSS helps prepare members to address these challenges. The first and foremost benefit the association provides is a comprehensive training program. Using this manual is one step in educating security personnel to the challenges of our profession.

As this edition goes to print, I am confident that the professional contributions and performance of each contributor will enhance the professionalism of healthcare security. I encourage each reader and student to move forward with his or her training, and I commend each of you for your desire to further your education. Through your professionalism, the healthcare institutions of our society are best able to function at their highest level of service.

Evelyn Meserve, CHPA
Editor in Chief

Contents

Contributors

How to Use This Book

Preface

Chapters

1. Introduction to Supervision
2. Supervisor Responsibilities
3. Employee Relations and Employee Appraisals
4. Authority and Control
5. Leadership
6. Handling Complaints and Grievances
7. Communication Skills in Supervision
8. Self-improvement
9. Civil Liability and the Supervisor
10. Safety and the Supervisor's Responsibilities
11. Budgeting and Cost Control
12. Principles of Customer Service
13. Professionalism and Ethics
14. Effective Crime Prevention Programs
15. Developing Training Plans and Programs
16. Security Operations
17. Planning for Emergency Management and Response
18. Supervisor Development

IAHSS Progressive Certification Program

Applications for the Supervisor Training Certification Examination

Chapter 1

Introduction to Supervision

Thomas A. Smith, CHPA, CPP

OBJECTIVES

After studying this chapter, the student should understand the following:

- Some of the elements of change and challenge facing healthcare security supervisors
- The demands of a healthcare security supervisor position
- Basic elements of and key terms used in healthcare security supervision
- Elements of successful healthcare security supervision

Will Rogers once said, "Good judgment comes from experience and a lot of that comes from bad judgment." Think about it. In your life, what experiences have had the biggest impact on your success? For starters, think about the experience you had as a child when you placed your hand on something hot, perhaps the oven or a coffee burner. The experience taught you pretty quickly the importance of listening to your mother when she screams and tells you to get away from something dangerous. Now think about those types of experiences as they apply to leadership and supervision.

As a security supervisor, your actions can result in liability to your organization and to you personally. False arrest or imprisonment, elopement of a patient who is a danger to himself or others, escape of a prisoner, employee grievances, or even death can result from security supervisors who over- or under-react to situations. These types of incidents can lead to loss of accreditation and severely damage your organization's reputation. Every day, incidents such as this are in the news and can be instructive to the security supervisor. Of course, learning from these kinds of experiences from a distance is always preferable.

Experiences play a major role in becoming a good supervisor. This manual provides you with the opportunity to learn from the experience of others. Supervision requires good judgment. It also requires hard work, modeling the behaviors you observe, education, training, and a heavy dose of experience. This chapter gives you a framework for further study of the materials in this book and resources for further outside study.

Change, Challenge, and Opportunities

No matter what business you work in change is constant. Anyone who has worked in healthcare for very long knows change seems to be "operating on steroids"; that is, change occurs so rapidly that keeping up with it is hard. In the past, patients came to the hospital; now healthcare services are provided near patient's homes through satellite clinics, mobile mammography units, pharmacies at local grocery stores, and health fairs at local schools and shopping malls. Healthcare has undergone rapid and continuous change for many years, with no end in sight.

In their book *Management Principles for Health Professionals*, Joan Liebler and Charles McConnell cite five major trends that continue to affect healthcare. These trends are listed below and discussed separately in the paragraphs that follow:

- Regulation of the healthcare industry
- Ongoing managed care mandates
- Restructuring of healthcare organizations through mergers, affiliations, and the virtual enterprise model
- Impact of technology
- Ongoing social and ethical factors

Regulation

Healthcare is one of the most regulated industries in the United States and Canada. State and federal governments strictly regulate healthcare facilities. The Centers for Medicare & Medicaid Services (CMS) is the US federal agency that administers

Medicare, Medicaid, and the State Children's Health Insurance Program. The Canada Health Act (CHA or the Act) is Canada's federal legislation for publicly funded healthcare insurance. The CHA establishes criteria and conditions related to insured health services and extended healthcare services that the provinces and territories must fulfill to receive the full federal cash contribution under the Canada Health Transfer (CHT). States, provinces, cities, and other local authorities also enact regulations directed at improving the administration, safety, and affordability of healthcare.

An example of regulations directly affecting healthcare security supervisors concerns the use of handcuffs. In 2004, the CMS published language excluding the use of handcuffs and other restraints by police or security officers working for healthcare facilities. This change in philosophy has caused many facilities to reconsider their deployment of handcuffs. Other items considered are CMS-published language on weapons and on the use of force.

Security supervisors must know the local regulatory requirements that affect how they do their jobs. Membership and active involvement in professional associations such as the IAHSS helps healthcare security professionals stay abreast of changes in the regulatory environment.

Managed Care

A primary aim of managed care systems is to control costs. Managed care systems usually rely on a primary care physician, who acts as a gatekeeper through whom the patient has to go to obtain other health services, such as specialty medical care, surgery, or physical therapy. Managed care plans strive to deliver efficient and cost-effective care. Recent trends have made this more challenging (e.g., rising age of the population, costly new technology, additional federal and state mandates, higher cost prescription drugs, and pressure from healthcare providers for higher fees).

Restructuring

If you have worked in healthcare for more than a year or two, you have probably lived through a merger, affiliation, or restructuring or witnessed one involving a local competitor. Restructuring usually holds risks and opportunities for the healthcare security supervisor. In the event the organization you are merging with has a different security model, your organization may have an opportunity to influence the other model. Alternatively, you may be more interested in the model used in the facility with which you are merging. In any case, paying close attention to and being aware of any opportunities that arise from corporate mergers is prudent.

Technology

Predicting when and how a new scientific or technological event will affect the security supervisory position is difficult. You must keep abreast of the changes affecting the healthcare security field. As new treatment options are more widely available and move closer to the patient bedside or home, staffing needs change and treatment locations change. In turn, security risks change and security needs change.

Medical Records Protection. In the United States, for example, the Health Insurance Portability and Accountability Act (HIPAA) requires organizations handling electronic health data to implement measures for controlling access to confidential medical information and protecting it against compromise and mis-use. Recently, courts have extended the law to cover paper records as well. Security supervisors should be familiar with the requirements of their employer for protecting medical records under this law.

Technology Skills. Security technology also has maintained pace with medical equipment. As hospitals apply more integrated electronic security measures, the need for different skills in security officers is evident. Many hospitals now have physical and/or electronic security specialists whose job is to help manage the growing security technology. Security officers now need computer skills and the ability to communicate effectively and to understand computer technology as it relates to security needs. The use of wireless handheld personal digital assistants, point-of-care computers, and so on will continue to grow, and supervisors and staff must become familiar with this aspect of their jobs to remain effective. Those who do not will find themselves searching for answers or possibly a job in another field.

Social and Ethical Factors
Social and ethical factors will have an important effect on the future of healthcare, and each has very specific impacts on security. Breakthroughs in genetic research and legislation regarding patient self-determination, abortion, and alternative therapies drive change. Security supervisors who maintain awareness of these factors as they relate to their local environment are better able to provide effective protection programs and more readily accepted as a part of the leadership team.

The Demands of a Security Supervisor Position

Supervisor positions in any healthcare department are usually quite challenging. A typical hospital administrative pyramid is shown on this page. Whether supervising a shift of employees in the lab, pharmacy, nutrition services, medical records, or security, supervisors are in the middle and serve as the link between the higher levels of administration and the employees at the base of the pyramid.

Typical Healthcare/Hospital Organizational Structure

Board of directors, trustees, or commissioners

President/chief executive officer (CEO)

Executive vice president/chief operating officer (COO)/ chief financial officer (CFO)

Vice presidents

Directors, department heads, managers

Supervisors

Employees

A common complicating factor is that the physicians (the people who can have a large impact on cash flow) do not typically fall within the pyramid. Physicians are often independent contractors; they may or may not be paid directly by the hospital. If a medical school is affiliated with the hospital, a separate reporting structure manages the relationship between the hospital, medical school, and patient care services.

Healthcare facilities with an affiliated medical school or university school of nursing or other teaching programs pose additional challenges for supervisors due to the added levels of communication and necessary management structures.

In addition, patients and visitors are usually under a great deal of stress because of an illness. As a result of this added stress, they sometimes act differently than they normally would. Minor inconveniences or limitations sometimes cause patients to become angry and irrational, and security staff is often called to respond.

Needless to say, healthcare facilities are complicated and supervisors in any department have a challenging job. Security supervisors have additional challenges because of the broad scope of duties and the impact those duties can have on patients and services provided by other departments.

For example, if a security officer forgets to open a parking lot gate on time and the patient/visitor lot fills up, patients do not show up for their appointments. Even if they show up, they may be upset and become management problems for the caregivers. Complaints soar and cash flow is affected due to missed or rescheduled appointments.

Many times, the smallest error or misjudgment committed by an officer is made into an example of incompetence by the security department. There are many similar examples of how security impacts every service and patient. The difficulty in this is that when things go well, people outside the security department seldom notice. This is the challenge of healthcare supervision.

Supervisors' Areas of Responsibility
In the book *Haimann's Healthcare Management*, Rose Dunn identifies four major dimensions, or four areas of responsibility, of every supervisory position. They are listed here, but note that their order does not equate to their importance.

- The supervisor must be responsible to the employees of the department.
- The supervisor must be responsible to his or her supervisor: typically, this is the security director or manager.
- The supervisor must act as a connecting link between the leadership of the department and the employees. The supervisor must accurately portray communications between the two groups and strive for clarity.
- The supervisor must maintain good working relationships with the department heads, leaders, and peer supervisors of all other departments and, not least of all, the physicians.

Customer Focus

Who are your most critical customers? Would it be the emergency department, psychiatry, physicians, outside law enforcement agencies? You need to know who your customers are and ensure your staff members are treating them like customers. Supervisors play an important role in keeping these customers coming back and using security's services. The best place to establish and maintain excellent customer relations is at the supervisor and employee level of the organizational chart. When things get kicked up the chain of command, communication can get foggy (let's just leave it at that).

Skills and Knowledge

In addition to these four dimensions, security supervisors must have good technical and professional skills to lead their areas of responsibility. You need technical knowledge of many areas of responsibility, including but not limited to the following:

- Human resource policies specific to your department
- Jurisdiction and use of force
- Patient restraint and elopement policies
- Emergency procedures
- Incident reporting procedures
- Related criminal and civil laws

- A healthy sense of humor
- Common sense

Basic Elements of Supervision

Are good supervisors made or chosen? The qualities that make up the essentials of supervision can relate to personal characteristics and skills (interpersonal, trade, technical). These qualities may include the following:

- Above-average leadership skills
- Team-building skills
- Good communications skills
- Excellent follow-through on projects and special assignments
- Regularly demonstrated interpersonal skills

Promotion to a supervisory position can be the result of superior on-the-job performance or based on similar past supervisory work experience. In either case, the personal leadership skills and attributes possessed by the supervisor are critical to the success of the operation and security function in healthcare.

Leadership Model

Just as your performance as a supervisor reflects on your manager, the performance of the security officers you supervise shows your leadership ability. In the past, many organizations have relied on the law enforcement model of organization, which is based on a paramilitary role. In these, there is a commander at the top, an assortment of other ranked leaders in the middle, and the rank-and-file officers at the operations level. The preferred model is changing, just as the expectations are changing for security departments. Present trends reflect these expectations, meaning that a different departmental model may exist at some institutions. A less military or police-like leadership style may be used. As a security supervisor, your leadership style must match the one used in the department and your organization.

Each institution has a specific set of values or beliefs that influences how the facility operates. You must know the culture of your organization, coupled with the attitudes prevalent in the organization, to be an effective supervisor. If your organization practices team-focused decision making, with employee participation in goal setting and monitoring, you need a supervisory style based on that culture. By the same token, if your department's practices have been comfortably based on a law enforcement model, which is supported by the organization's management, your values may reflect this style of leadership. Your supervisory style should reflect the values desired by your organization. You can strengthen this style with the personal leadership traits you bring to the job.

The Transition to Supervisor

When a person is selected to become a supervisor or team leader, the person's qualifications and past performance are usually the basis of the decision. Transitioning from rank-and-file employee to supervisor can be challenging and sometimes difficult. Supervisors often have to take on a new perspective about the work world and their role and responsibilities in it.

Often, a manager chooses a supervisor based on a variety of qualifications and a personal "fit." The definition of fit has much to do with the personalities on the management or leadership team as well as the new supervisor's ability to fit into this team. Anticipating exactly how you should act as a new supervisor is sometimes difficult, as is understanding how these actions will meet management's expectations of you. However, you need to remember that your selection to the role of supervisor is based on a level of trust that management has in your ability to get the job done.

In his book *Life's Greatest Lessons*, Hal Urban provides an excellent template for being a good supervisor. He writes, "You can do many things I suggest here—have a positive attitude, form good habits, laugh, be thankful, set goals, motivate yourself, work hard, be self-disciplined, use time wisely, etc.— but you'll never be truly successful unless everything you do is undergirded with honesty and integrity." *The most important factor in being a healthcare security supervisor is honesty and integrity.* Beyond that, here are a few more suggestions:

- Be flexible. When things do not go according to plan, adjust and overcome.
- Before you attempt to tell others how to run their shift, department, or other service, make sure you have your own ship in order.
- Have a positive attitude about your department, your organization, and your profession. No one wants to be around someone who is always complaining. Work to fix the problems and do not worry about things out of your span of control or influence.
- Be technically proficient. Make sure you can do what you are asking your employees to do.
- Take advantage of leadership training and quality improvement projects at your institution. The time you spend with other supervisors and managers helps you develop supporting relationships that pay off when you need to work on an important issue related to your security or safety responsibilities.
- Find a mentor with leadership qualities you wish to emulate. Mentors can not only teach, but also help keep leaders firmly grounded and directed during the critical early days of their management roles.
- If you are solidly successful in your role, be a mentor.
- Find time for professional development. Get involved in your local IAHSS chapter. Ensure your team has opportunities for professional development.
- Stay in touch with your customers. Make sure you know what they want and then ensure you are providing quality service.
- Stay abreast of changes in your local environment and the industry.
- There is an old saying, "Do not expect what you don't inspect." More often than not, that is true—not because employees do not want to or do not care to perform their tasks, but simply because of human frailty. Ensure your staff is doing what they

are supposed to do (e.g., security checks, light inspections, parking lot patrols).

- If you disagree with your manager, take it up with him or her. Do not air these differences in front of your subordinates.

- Have a succession plan. One way to streamline future promotions is to develop your replacement. Make sure you have people you manage who can step in when you are not there. This makes you more available for other assignments and future promotions.

Conclusion

As you move forward in your supervisory role, you should remain adaptive and continue to build on your knowledge. This chapter stressed that supervisors come from a variety of backgrounds and possess varied degrees of leadership skills. The security supervisor himself or herself is the engine that drives change and personal success. In *Superior Supervision: The 10% Solution*, Raymond Loen wrote, "Your ability to create constructive change can be the greatest single indicator of your supervisory performance." Your career path will have many opportunities for personal and professional growth. This path can be slow or fast, and much of this depends on you. A supervisor's growth, self-learning, and development can speed this process while building the needed self-assurance and self-respect required to be an effective leader.

The opportunities ahead for healthcare security supervisors can be summed up in the words of a Chinese proverb: "The journey of one thousand miles starts with the first step." By understanding the supervisor's role, the healthcare organization's expectations, and the steps necessary to make your transition into that role, your journey will be a fulfilling and happy one.

Key Terms and Abbreviations in Healthcare

The following are terms and abbreviations healthcare security supervisors should know.

Term or Abbreviation	Meaning
Accreditation	Hospitals are accredited or non-accredited.
FTE	Full-time equivalent. Used in developing budgets and schedules. Someone who works 40 hours in a one-week pay period or 80 hours in a two-week pay period.
CMS	Centers for Medicare & Medicaid Services (CMS). US federal agency that administers Medicare, Medicaid, and the State Children's Health Insurance Program. CMS has very specific regulations affecting the duties of security officers involved in patient restraint and other patient-related duties.
Healthcare facility (HCF)	For the purposes of the Guidelines from Premises Security, 2006 edition (Guideline #730 from the National Fire Protection Association), the term means a facility used for providing medical service or treatment simultaneously to four or more patients... • who are primarily incapable of self-preservation due to physical or mental limitations or • who are undergoing treatment or under anesthesia, which renders such patients incapable of taking actions under emergency conditions without assistance from others.
HIPAA	Health Insurance Portability and Accountability Act
The Joint Commission	In early 2007, the Joint Commission on Accreditation of Healthcare Organizations shortened its name to The Joint Commission. The Joint Commission provides accreditation and certification programs to various types of healthcare organizations.

Bibliography

Meserve, E. (ed.). 2007. *Basic Training Manual for Healthcare Security Officers*, 4th ed. Glendale Heights, Ill: International Association for Healthcare Security and Safety.

Centers for Medicare & Medicaid Services. 21 May 2004. State Operations Manual. On the Internet: www.cms.hhs.gov/manuals/Downloads/som107ap_a_hospitals.pdf. Accessed 15 Jun 2007.

Dunn, R. T. 2007. *Haimann's Healthcare Management*, 8th ed. Davis, J. (ed.). Chicago: Health Administration Press.

Health Canada. 13 Oct 2005. Canada Health Act. On the Internet: www.hc-sc.gc.ca/hcs-sss/medi-assur/overview-apercu/index_e.html. Accessed 15 Jun 2007.

Liebler, J. and C. McConnell. 2004. *Management Principles for Health Professionals*, 4th ed. Sudbury, Mass: Jones and Bartlett Publishers.

Loen, R. O. 1994. *Superior Supervision: The 10% Solution.* New York: Lexington Books.

Urban, H. 2003. *Life's Greatest Lessons*, 4th ed. New York: Simon and Schuster, Inc.

Vijayan, J. 15 Jun 2007. HIPAA audit at hospital riles healthcare IT. Computer World. On the Internet: www.computerworld.com/action/article.do?command=viewArticleBasic&articleId=9024921. Accessed 18 Jun 2007.

Study and Review Questions

1. What always stays constant regardless of where you work?

    A. Change

    B. Pressure

    C. Attitude

    D. Work conditions

2. What is the goal of managed care systems?

    A. To increase costs

    B. To control costs

    C. To increase documentation

    D. To decrease documentation

3. Which category in the institution's organizational chart best describes line officers' position?

    A. Board of directors

    B. Vice presidents

    C. Employees

    D. Chief executive officer

4. What is the most important factor in being a security supervisor?

    A. Communication skills

    B. Professional appearance

    C. Writing skills

    D. Honesty and integrity

Chapter 2

Supervisor Responsibilites

Alan J. Butler, CHPA

OBJECTIVES

After studying this chapter, the student should understand the following:

- Certain skills and talents contribute to being a good supervisor
- Personnel are the department's most valuable resource
- Supervisors fulfill various roles; two especially important ones are advocating for employees and advocating for the organization
- Supervisors have two kinds of responsibilities: those involving personnel and those involving tasks
- Supervisors must be diligent about documentation, as they are responsible for a variety of written communications
- Supervisors must set and apply boundaries that protect the organization and the security officers
- Ensuring the "little things" are in place for employees allows them to concentrate on their work
- Problems need to be addressed by supervisors, not ignored

Organizational Structure

The size of an organization often determines the security department's structure. The larger the organization is the more likely security will have multiple levels of supervision. Often when there are multiple levels of supervision, front-line supervisors concentrate on the needs of a single shift. In smaller organizations, one supervisor may be responsible for the entire patrol function. Quality time with your staff is important. The more spread out they are, across multiple shifts, the more difficulty you will have finding time with them. Consider how your organization's structure affects your interactions with your staff.

The security function is important in a healthcare organization's overall mission to provide a safe environment. The organization determines to whom the healthcare security department reports. Having a champion for the security cause as close as possible to the top executive of the organization may very well determine the success of the department and, quite importantly, its funding. Regardless of the reporting structure, you want to maintain a positive, open, and professional relationship with the person to whom you report.

A Good Supervisor

Being a good supervisor requires a number of skills and talents. Being a good or even a great officer does not necessarily mean you will be an effective supervisor. The foundations from which you operate and the manner in which you respond to various supervisory challenges depend on your ability to do the following:

- Make sound, value-based judgments
- Be honest, fair, and ethical
- Listen with genuine interest
- Be accountable—especially when you make a mistake
- Make tough decisions
- Make timely decisions
- Display personal and professional confidence

Creating Balance

Perhaps most importantly, a good supervisor is one who can create balance. The supervisor position is where the "rubber meets the road." Supervisors are pulled in many directions, and their ability to find balance often determines their success. You must be balanced in the way you interact with staff, subordinates, superiors, and the organization. You must also recognize that your employees need to balance their work and personal lives. Although individuals may juggle their top priorities, recognize that work often comes below significant personal and family matters. Good supervisors understand how this affects staff and the work environment.

Security's Most Valuable Asset: Your Employees

This is not hard to figure out, yet every day in security departments across the country supervisors, managers, and directors fail to recognize who makes most of the critical (in-the-moment) security decisions in their organization. It is the front-line security officer. In most cases, an officer makes a dozen critical decisions before you or anyone else in leadership has time to respond to a call for assistance.

You need look no further than your annual operating budget to witness the impact of your staff. In most cases, labor and labor-related costs amount to more than 93 percent of all security operating budgets.

Building a Supportive Environment

Your first job is to make sure that staff members have the tools they need to do their work, the training necessary to make good decisions, and a work environment that allows them to do their job.

Actively engaged employees are those who can tell you they enjoy the work they do, where they do it, and those with whom they work. Work should be a place where employees like to come, a place where they feel they belong and can contribute. Creating this type of work environment is easier said than done, but certainly doable.

Start with trust, a five-letter word that has more impact on one's ability to successfully supervise than any other in the dictionary. Some of the most important lessons on trust are these:

- Learn to start from the position that you trust people until they give you a reason not to trust them, rather than requiring them to earn your trust first.
- Recognize that the above statement does not apply to how your staff will treat you. You have to earn their trust. Your consistent actions over time are the best indicators of your trustworthiness.
- You cannot have hidden agendas. Say what you will do and do what you said you would.
- Build an environment of trust by soliciting, listening to, and acting on staff suggestions.
- Trust yourself and have confidence in your ability to do the job. Make good, fair, and timely decisions. Stand behind other good decisions, and never be afraid to admit you made a mistake.

Supervisors Are Advocates

Advocating for Your Employees

The supervisor is often the link between staff and the organization. A good supervisor knows an employee's strengths as well as the opportunities that person has for improvement. You interact with an employee on a level that many in the organization never see. Do your best to put employees in situations where they are most likely to be successful. In doing so, you create a win-win situation for the employee and the organization.

Supervisors also represent a line of communication from the employee to department leadership. You need to recognize which information is meant to stay with you and which is meant to move elsewhere in the organization. Your communication must be completely unbiased and accurate. Understanding these critical points helps develop trust between staff and supervisor.

Advocating for the Organization

As much as you are an advocate for the employee, you are equally, if not more, an advocate for the organization. For many beginning supervisors, this is a new role. You understand the employee point of view because you were one, but the organizational piece is new. Now you are the link between the organization and the employee—for example, regarding issues raised in the weekly staff meeting, a policy review, or a post order change. In meetings, you represent both the employee and the organization, but in the end you must first do what is best for the organization. Your viewpoint in staff meetings and your communication with staff must strongly align with the organization's direction.

If you are unwilling to stand behind the organization, this job is not for you. This does not mean that you cannot disagree. Rather, you must fight the right battles in the right forum. Then, when the door opens and the smoke settles, you must toe the company line because that is what is best for the organization. A simple rule of thumb is what is good for the team or the organization wins out over what is good for the individual.

Two Sides to Supervision

Although there are many responsibilities within the role of supervisor, most work falls in two distinct areas:

- Personnel
- Tasks

Personnel Matters

Among your responsibilities regarding personnel, the following are key items. The paragraphs that follow provide more detail on each.

- Hiring, training, and retraining
- Giving recognition
- Coaching and mentoring
- Evaluating performance
- Taking disciplinary action and terminating employees
- Dealing flexibly with employees' personal issues

Why is it so important to stay on top of issues related to personnel? Because supervisors matter to employees. The authors of *First, Break All the Rules* make the following observation when it comes to why employees stay or leave a business.

Their research suggests that although employee-focused initiatives (e.g., vacation time, daycare, profit sharing, training) are a consideration, the employee's immediate manager is *more* important. The supervisor defines and pervades the work environment, they explain:

- When a supervisor "sets clear expectations, knows you, trusts you, and invests in you, then you can forgive the company its lack of a profit-sharing program."

- "If your relationship with your manager is fractured, then no amount of in-chair massaging or company-sponsored dog walking will persuade you to stay and perform."

Working for a great manager in an old-fashioned company, they write, is better than working for a terrible manager in a company offering an enlightened, employee-focused culture. Keep this in mind as you go about your work.

Hiring, Training, and Retaining. Recruiting, interviewing, and hiring the right people are the starting point of building a good team. Good supervisors recognize the importance of finding the right people. New employees have to be suitable in two critical areas: they have to be able to do the job and, almost as important, they have to fit. An employee has to fit philosophically with what your organization stands for and has to fit on your team. Nothing rocks the boat worse than a bad fit.

Once you find the right person, you have to train this employee in the ways of your organization and your profession. Make sure you have a good training program in place for new recruits and that you are an active participant in that program.

Finally, since you have invested considerable time and money into these individuals, you must work to retain them. Some recruits catch on fast, but most take a while to fully understand the job. The longer they stay, the better the return on your organization's investment.

Recognition. Although not every employee likes to be recognized in the same way, almost all employees like to be recognized. Find out what works best for your staff and then find opportunities to recognize their accomplishments. Whether you recognize an employee at a shift briefing in front of the group or through a personal letter sent to the employee's home, giving recognition is important. Ensure the recognition you give is timely and genuine. If you are just "going through the motions" so you can say you recognize staff, your insincerity will have the greater impact. Real recognition, given correctly, makes an impact and helps build individual as well as team morale.

Coaching and Mentoring. Having the opportunity to grow and contribute at work is important to good employees. These employees look for opportunities to contribute. As a supervisor, you must recognize what various staff members are good at and then work to put them in situations where they can flourish. Also, you must recognize where opportunities for improvement exist and look for ways to facilitate your employees' professional growth.

Part of being a good coach and mentor is recognizing that everyone learns differently. Some people need only to read about a topic once before applying the information. Others may have to read, see, and do before the lesson is learned. Aim to understand what works best for each person you teach.

Evaluations. Evaluating an employee's performance is not something that occurs once a year. Evaluations are an ongoing process. The next chapter is about evaluations, but in understanding your responsibilities you must be aware that documenting employee performance is an essential, everyday process.

Many good supervisors log key interactions and observations related to their employees' performance. Sometimes this consists of just brief notes in their file. By itself, one note may mean very little, but in the greater context of an employee's overall performance, these observations might mean more. Keep in mind that this type of documentation is not restricted to poor performance issues; include observations of good or outstanding performance as well.

Your ongoing, day-to-day documentation makes annual evaluations much easier. From it, you can cite examples rather than make general comments about performance.

Discipline and Terminations. Having to discipline or terminate an employee is a task every supervisor dreads, but an important part of the supervisory role. Seasoned supervisors will tell you that avoiding this type of confrontation by doing nothing is the worst thing you can do. Ignoring a serious problem is not fair to the employee, who many times deserves an opportunity to fix what is broken. It is also unfair to the rest of the team, who look to you to create a fair and balanced workplace.

As with performance evaluations, you must precede this type of action with timely and accurate documentation. Gather unbiased and truthful supporting documentation. Make sure that, regardless of the action taken, you have documentation that protects the organization in case of litigation.

Finally, recognize that sometimes a termination is the best course for all involved. You may not feel that way at the time you terminate someone, but if you are a fair supervisor, you know you have arrived at this point for a reason. In concert with your supporting partners—human resources personnel and your manager—you are going to do what is best for the organization, your department, and possibly the individual.

Personal Issues. You cannot separate employees' personal lives from their work lives. How a person acts at work is often directly affected by events at home and vice versa. You will often have to deal with work effects of issues from employees' personal lives. Following the caveats below helps you have satisfied, productive employees.

- Recognize that employees are generally going to view situations from their own perspectives and think first about what works for and is good for them

- Be flexible in dealing with employees' personal issues

- Be willing to sit down with employees and listen to their issues
- Identify resources that may help

Yes, employees generally function best with established boundaries and guidelines, but they need to know that you will at least listen and, when possible, be flexible when an issue arises. This is especially pertinent in scheduling and issues that impact activities outside work.

You will not always have a solution, but may be able to direct them to other resources. Regardless, effective listening is part of the supervisory role. To the extent that you are a good listener, you will be rewarded with a healthy and productive staff.

For many years, employers tried to keep personal life issues out of the workplace. The belief was that employees were somehow supposed to leave all personal baggage at the door and concentrate only on work. Unfortunately, that does not work. The best supervisors and the best organizations recognize that, when it comes to staff, you get the whole person. That often includes personal issues. Generally speaking, you will do well to take at least a casual interest in the personal lives of your staff.

Task Matters

In addition to having significant responsibilities regarding personnel, supervisors attend to several key tasks. The following are discussed in the paragraphs that follow:

- Documentation
- Scheduling
- Budgets
- Other assigned duties
- Policies and procedures
- Investigations
- Uniforms and equipment

Documentation. Paperwork is so important in the supervisory role. Your paperwork reflects who you are. The professionalism of your work as well as that of your organization is usually evident from your paperwork. Often, ability to communicate in writing determines an individual's success as a supervisor. The documentation types listed below are common to everyday security work:

- Incident reports
- Memos—internal and external
- Policies and procedures
- Investigations
- Personnel-related documentation
- Employee recognition

These written materials are all different, yet equally important. In an incident report, a missed step or a bad time sequence can mean the difference between a conviction and an acquittal. Using "there" instead of "their" in a memo suggests you do not proof your work, which may cause someone to wonder what other types of mistakes you make. Paperwork is important and a big part of your everyday job.

Scheduling. No task you perform may be more important than preparing the schedule. The schedule must, first, work for your organization and, second, be fair and equitable for your staff. Providing your organization with adequate staffing has major implications for the safety of patients, visitors, and staff. The adequacy of staffing may later be challenged in court, so getting it right is important. Balancing between organizational staffing goals and personnel needs is a challenge supervisors face each day. Having well-defined guidelines for selecting and receiving regularly scheduled days off, holidays, and vacation time goes a long way toward keeping staff happy. Try to avoid last-minute changes in employee schedules; these aggravate employees. Give as much lead time as possible when making scheduling decisions.

Budgets. Although you may not be asked to prepare the budget, you will certainly have input. Generally speaking, departments only get one chance to present operational and capital budgets so getting it right the first time is important.

A majority of security's operational budget is for costs associated with staff wages, salaries, and benefits. Therefore, being able to justify staffing needs is important. Using industry and community standards as well as benchmarking studies helps. Many times, though, staffing is particular to the organization. You must consider factors such as the following:

- *Size of Facility, Types of Services Offered:* Some services require more attention from security (e.g., in-house psychiatry, labor and delivery, postpartum care, pediatrics, the emergency department)
- *Geographic Setting:* Urban or rural
- *Trauma Level of the Emergency Department*
- *Crime Rate in the Community:* Especially the area immediately surrounding the hospital

The other major portion of the operational budget is equipment costs. How to manage annual equipment needs is best understood at the point where the products and equipment are used. In other words, do not be afraid to seek input from your staff regarding the supplies and equipment necessary to run the department. Their input alongside yours will go a long way toward budget preparation and resource utilization.

The budget should not be a secret. The more that staff and especially front-line supervision know about the budget and the cost of running a department the more likely they are to respect and manage daily costs. This also creates an important sense of team.

With few exceptions, security departments do not generate revenue. Therefore, every penny spent on security is truly an investment in preventing what might happen. Good security administrators track and validate the cost-benefit of services they provide. Some data are easy to identify (e.g., the money saved by catching a thief stealing computers). Other benefits are harder to identify, but just as important (e.g., crime prevention and personal safety efforts).

Other Duties as Assigned. Every boss includes this category somewhere in the job description. Even if you do not see it, it is there. These duties could include anything. For example, you may be given a last-minute project requiring crime statistics related to emergency department activity or asked to build a database for new security incident report writing software. Regardless of the project, these assignments are one way you contribute to the growth of the department as well as your own personal and professional growth.

When assigned a special project, be sure to understand fully the expectations and time line; if they are not clear, ask for further explanation. Going to your boss with the completed project only to find that it is not exactly what they were looking for is indeed disappointing. Managing projects is an important piece of the supervisor's job and certainly something on which you are evaluated.

Policies and Procedures. Most everybody hates the thought of writing policy, but this task does not have to be difficult. You do not need to create policy from scratch. Hospital security departments have been around for quite some time. Little that you do in your organization has not been done elsewhere. Network with other organizations. Go to the IAHSS Web site and review sample policies. Use what you can and make adjustments where needed.

Nowadays, much is often left to staff interpretation and discretion. Despite all the "gray areas," recognize that boundaries are still needed. Policies and procedures are written to protect the organization and the officers. The boundaries we create—through policy and procedure, written guidelines, and established practices—provide this protection. You are part of the process that helps establish (1) the ground rules and (2) the consistency under which your officers make these daily decisions.

Investigations. Sometimes a simple incident report turns into an investigation. As a supervisor, you may have to decide how much time you or your staff can devote, which investigations are within your realm of expertise, and which ones need to be handed off. A few other things to remember are mentioned here.

First, if you need to go outside your organization for help on an investigation, you can pretty much bet that whatever happens from that point forward is outside your control. This is neither good nor bad; it just is.

Second, if you are able to handle the investigation within the organization, recognize that managers of other departments may need to be involved. In matters that involve employees, the security department is usually an extension of the human resource function. Everything you discover will probably be turned over to them for final disposition.

Keep in mind that giving department managers input into the final disposition makes them more likely to be up front with you and use security as a resource. No good manager likes having someone else handle their personnel matters. To the extent that you give that control back at the end of the investigation, you cultivate a relationship in which managers are more likely to work with you rather than work around you.

Uniforms and Equipment. In security, uniforms and equipment are the everyday items every officer needs to do the job. Gallup researchers determined that there are 12 questions that measure the core elements needed to attract, focus, and keep the most talented employees (Wagner 2007). One of the most pertinent questions is this: Do I have the materials and equipment I need to do my work right?

Minor as it seems, when employees lack the things they need to do their job correctly, the negative impact on their work performance is huge. Stay in tune with their needs and make sure they have what they need in a timely manner. If your employees are asking for items they have run out of, you have been remiss. Yes, the little things are significant.

Keeping an Eye on the Little Things

For years, good supervisors have known one simple secret to keeping employees content: take care of the little things. Every one of us wishes we had a person to take care of the "little things" that affect us. We would like someone to make sure all the little, everyday things are taken care of so we can concentrate on the more important parts of our job. To make operations run smoothly, supervisors attend to little things. Doing so keeps these things little.

Enabling Employees to Focus on Work

As it pertains to your staff, being responsible for the little things starts with you. You do not have to do it all, but you need to know that the little things are getting done. For example:

- Schedules completed well in advance
- Uniforms ordered on time
- Batteries for flashlights in stock
- Spare radio microphones on hand, just in case

Any one of these everyday issues that is out of place, not in stock, or addressed at only the last minute forces your employees to take their minds off business and concentrate on one of life's little aggravations.

Keeping Problems Small

Whenever possible, "keep things little." That is, address problems as they arise. Do not procrastinate or wait for problems to go away on their own. With time, problems just get bigger. Unfortunately, when it comes to problems, very often you cannot delegate the fix. Certainly, you can seek advice from others, but you have to be able to exercise the responsibility associated with your position. Your staff and boss expect that you will make decisions. They even know and expect that not all of those decisions will involve answers they want to hear. Believe it or not, they are all right with that. They will have much more respect for you for making the decision and standing by it than if you make no decision at all.

Conclusion

Good supervisors do not happen by accident. They are a product of hard work, tremendous patience, continuous learning, and a genuine commitment to staff. The responsibilities outlined in this chapter are meant to guide you in your endeavors to develop a long and fruitful relationship with your staff and employer.

Bibliography

Buckingham, M. and C. Coffman. 1999. *First, Break All The Rules.* New York: Simon & Schuster, Inc. pp. 28 and 34.

Wagner, R., F. Drumond and J. K. Harter. 8 Mar 2007. The 12 elements of great managing (sidebar to Why employees need the right equipment). *Gallup Management Journal.* On the Internet: http://gmj.Gallup.com/content/26773/2/Why-Employees-Need-the-Right-Equipment.aspx. Accessed 4 Jun 2007.

Study and Review Questions

1. Who makes most of the critical security decisions in the organization?

A. Security manager

B. Security supervisor

C. Security officer

D. Security director

2. For whom do supervisors advocate?

A. Employees and the organization

B. Employees and the department

C. The department and organization

D. Employees and supervisors

3. What are the two distinct sides of a supervisor's work?

A. Personnel and administration

B. Administration and tasks

C. Personnel and coaching

D. Personnel and tasks

4. Which of these is not a task assigned to the supervisor?

A. Documentation

B. Coaching and mentoring

C. Scheduling

D. Budget

5. What is the simple secret to keeping employees content?

A. Change the schedule often

B. Have an open-door policy

C. Take care of the little things

D. Be friends with staff

Chapter 3

Employee Relations and Employee Appraisals

Chris Leibfried, CHPA

OBJECTIVES

After studying this chapter, the student should understand the following:

- The elements of employee relations
- The value of employee recognition and how it fosters motivation
- The purpose of employee appraisals
- Effective management of progressive discipline
- The value of an employee assistance program

Employee Relations

Employee relations are the employer-employee relationship that promotes morale, motivation, and productivity. The goal of employee relations is to prevent and resolve employee problems that are a product of or affect employee work situations.

Employee Orientation

Management has the responsibility to provide employees with a clear interpretation of the organization's mission, vision, policies, and goals. Employees should learn of these fundamental objectives during their initial orientation. The orientation should especially make clear each of the following:

- The conduct expected of employees
- Non-discrimination and non-harassment protocols (As a matter of policy, the organization should strictly prohibit retaliation against anyone reporting discrimination or harassment or cooperating with an investigation.)

Periodic Meetings

An effective mechanism for continually promoting effective employer-employee relations is a monthly meeting. A town hall model is an ideal form to foster the objectives. The following parties should attend:

- ***Management Representatives:*** Representatives of the administration, nursing leadership, human resources, quality management, and security should participate.
- ***Employee Representatives:*** Representatives from each clinical and non-clinical department should attend. Their role is to (1) represent and provide departmental input and (2) provide feedback to their departments.
- ***Security Management:*** All or any part of the security management team may attend. These meetings are a great opportunity for the security supervisor to pass on information and hear employee concerns.

Communicating the Positive

A positive and productive opening from management incorporates what is new and good relevant to the department of interest. This type of opening communication solicits employees to give positive feedback. The following are examples of positive developments that may be related during this portion of the meeting:

- Press Ganey scores
- New services
- New locations of offices and services
- Construction projects
- Promotions
- Recognition

Identifying Potential Negatives

Employees are given the opportunity to share concerns, problems, or processes that are potential inhibitors in their work environment. Management must then respond to the identified inhibitors and formulate corrective actions for legitimate problems. The employees should be part of the process of creating corrective action plans. As appropriate, some of this problem solving must occur after the meeting rather than during it.

Reporting and Solutions
Management records the minutes and distributes them in a timely manner. The minutes summarize the following:
- The positive news reported and the positive comments made
- Concerns, complaints, and issues discussed
- Planned corrective actions

Communications
The minutes and issues are then shared at departmental meetings. This further fosters positive employer-employee communications to all first-line employees.

According to Russell Colling in *Hospital and Healthcare Security*, "Today's officers want more input into decisions that affect them than their predecessors did. If management fails to listen to employees, is unresponsive to their needs, or fails to deliver deserved recognition, employees will not perform in a satisfactory manner."

Employee Recognition

Focusing on employee recognition develops an atmosphere that promotes teamwork, cooperation, innovation, and appreciation for individual and collective contribution. With this focus, the workforce becomes more highly motivated to "go the extra distance" for patients, visitors, and staff. As a supervisor, you have a critical role in recognizing the contributions of your employees. What you do ultimately affects productivity and morale within your department. The sidebar outlines the goals of employee recognition efforts.

Goals of Employee Recognition
- Reinforce desired behaviors in the workplace
- Improve staff morale and satisfaction
- Increase productivity
- Promote teamwork
- Reward positive attitudes
- Deter negative attitudes
- Demonstrate value by the organization
- Increase loyalty to the organization
- Decrease turnover
- Create satisfied employees who contribute to satisfied patients and favorable Press Ganey scores

---

The following are examples of employee recognition programs (North Shore–Long Island Jewish Health System 2006, ERP). Each of these is discussed separately in the paragraphs that follow.
- "Applause" cards
- Service excellence awards
- Employee recognition awards
- Professional recognition weeks or months
- Other employee relations activities

"Applause" Cards
You and your organization can use thank-you cards to recognize positive inter-personal behavior among employees. Doing so builds teamwork and camaraderie and demonstrates appreciation and acknowledgement for a job well done. Applause cards can be given from a colleague to a peer, from a manager to a staff member, and from a staff member to a manager.

Service Excellence Awards
You and your organization can give special awards to recognize individuals who demonstrate outstanding

behavior with regard to service, teamwork, caring, and initiative. The awards may be given monthly, quarterly, or yearly.

Employee Recognition Awards

An awards ceremony for outstanding performance and continued service is another way to honor employees. Employees can, for example, be recognized for their years of service to the organization (e.g., in five-year increments).

Professional Recognition Weeks (or Months)

Your organization can sponsor a week-long or month-long celebration focusing on the contributions of individual professional groups (e.g., nursing, social work, physical therapy, security).

Other Employee Relations Activities

Consider other activities your organization can offer to improve employee relations. For example:

- Holiday parties for employees or their children
- Employee barbecues, luncheons, and picnics
- Inter- and intra-facility sports events

Employee Appraisals

The purpose of an appraisal is to evaluate how each employee's performance measures up to the requirements of the position. For accreditation, The Joint Commission mandates that employee performance evaluations be completed and include the following (The Joint Commission 2006; HR 1.20, 3.10, and 3.20):

- *Planning:* Determine if staff qualifications are consistent with the employee's job responsibilities
- *Assessing Competence:* Assess, demonstrate, and maintain the staff's competence to perform job responsibilities
- *Periodic Evaluations of Performance*

Ongoing Process

Understand that appraisals are not done just once a year. Rather, this is a continuing process involving the tasks noted in the sidebar. If you omit any step, you are not using the appraisal process effectively for employee development.

> **Employee Appraisal: An Ongoing Process**
> - Observe the work being performed
> - Evaluate the results
> - Maintain records
> - Communicate with the employee
> - Train the employee
> - Observe performance again

Conducting an orientation appraisal ensures the new employee understands the job, the department's expectations and goals, and the healthcare organization's expectations and goals. You can use a checklist or an appraisal for this and cover all "must know" information. Typically, it is best to complete an orientation appraisal at 30 days and again at 90 days of employment, after a probationary period. Throughout the employee's employment, you then have many appropriate opportunities to evaluate performance and provide individual feedback and guidance. The following is a common approach:

- *New Hire Appraisal:* Conduct an informal and constructive appraisal with the new employee. Continue on a day-to-day basis, whether favorable or unfavorable.
- *Probationary Appraisal:* Complete a formal evaluation at the end of the probationary period. Recommend continued employment or termination.
- *Ongoing Informal Review:* Continue informal performance reviews on an ongoing basis with retained employees until the next formal appraisal.
- *Formal Review:* Define goals for improvement and employee development.

Be aware that you must appropriately document all phases of both informal and formal evaluations.

Developmental Appraisals

Traditionally, appraisals have emphasized how the organization views the employee's performance opportunities for transfer/promotion and training decisions. This traditional appraisal method relies primarily on a past performance methodology. Usually, employees are evaluated based on these appraisals. One disadvantage of this approach is that numerical rankings encourage employees to compare themselves to peers.

Conversely, a developmental appraisal uses traditional appraisal components but incorporates a structure of communication between the employee and management. Management then has a means to clarify its expectations of the employee. An appraisal that focuses on development emphasizes the organization's interest in employee development for retention. Most importantly, this approach encourages an opportunity to formally indicate the direction and level of the employee's ambition, without a ranking.

In the table, you see one organization's tool for communicating its expectations and conducting its evaluations via a developmental appraisal. This tool describes 14 competencies, 11 of which apply to staff members such as security officers (the other 3—shaded in gray—pertain to department heads and front-line managers, including supervisors). Each desired competency is listed (in this case, predominantly in alphabetical order) and defined. For each competency, the tool describes what it looks like when an employee meets the criteria, does not meet the criteria, or exceeds the criteria.

At the appraisal, both the officer and the supervisor work from this list. The supervisor reviews the applicable competencies and solicits feedback from the employee. The goal is a dialogue. The supervisor listens for how the employee views his or her individual performance in each area. The employee's responses create opportunities for more dialogue. The result is a collective evaluation by supervisor and employee.

This example shows how the developmental appraisal process fosters effective, objective communications. The traditional process, in comparison, is the product of only the supervisor's perception and a numerical ranking of employees.

Sample of a Developmental Appraisal Tool

Criteria	Does Not Meet	Meets	Exceeds
Accountability/Ownership Takes responsibility for resolving problems	Passes the responsibility for assigned tasks to others or denies responsibility for assigned work.	Takes responsibility for resolving problems. Is proactive and consistent.	Becomes recognized local authority on problem resolution and has available substantial solutions. Teaches others to *see it, own it, solve it, and do it*.
Adaptability Changes based on business needs	Displays reluctance to alter own behavior based on business needs.	Changes behavior or action based on business needs.	Changes organization practice based on business direction and future needs.

Caring Shows compassion to others	Shows indifference to others or is inconsistent in showing compassion.	Shows compassion to others on a consistent basis, regardless of background or appearance.	Shows compassion to others. Works to systematize practices that foster caring throughout the health system.
Patient First Exceeds patient and customer expectations	Fails to satisfy patient or customer expectations.	Meets patient or customer expectations and consistently reaches out.	Exceeds patient or customer expectations by setting new service standards for their department, unit, or facility.
Engagement Shows up on time, ready to work	Displays indifference for proper work preparation and frequent tardiness/absence in attendance.	Shows up on time consistently, ready to work and focused on results.	Displays extraordinary productivity in work results, especially under pressure.
Excellence Pursues excellence with passion and promotes quality	Fails to promote quality in all aspects of job and does not seek to improve.	Determines business objectives and assesses the state of excellence against personal objectives.	Shows passion for the job. Assesses job scenarios to determine strengths and opportunities for improvement for self and others.
Execution Completes all work accurately	Fails to complete work consistently.	Completes all work accurately and consistently.	Completes all work flawlessly. Sets an example to others. Sets stretch-goals for self and consistently achieves these goals.
Innovation Brings new ideas to the job	Displays indifference to more productive ways to do job.	Brings new ideas to the job regularly.	Brings new ideas to the job and impacts other areas positively in adopting new practices.
Organizational Awareness Understands and learns formal and informal decision-making structures and relationships in the organization	Lacks in understanding formal and informal organizational structures and relationships. Does not adapt to organizational climate and culture.	Uses the formal hierarchy of the organization to get things done. Understands the chain of command, positional power, rules and regulations, policies, and procedures.	Identifies the real decision makers and has the ability to predict how new events will affect individuals and groups within the organization. Recognizes and uses ongoing power and political relationships within the constituencies with a clear sense of organizational impact.

Talent Development Builds the breadth and depth of the organization's human capability and professionalism	Does not express positive expectations of others or support ongoing development. Does not act as a developer of talent.	Makes positive comments regarding others' development future. Provides short-term, task-oriented instruction and promotes ongoing development.	Supports top performers and takes personal interest in coaching and mentoring top performers. Grows middle performers. Addresses low performers and takes action.
Team Leadership Sees oneself as a leader of others	Does not manage team meetings well. Fails to keep a constant staff. Does not promote team effectiveness.	Takes interest in forming a team that possesses balanced capabilities to setting its mission, values, and norms. Acts as a strong team player with peers.	Manages team meetings well, promotes team effectiveness, and is a role model for leadership. Holds the team accountable individually and as a group for results. Is a team builder among their peer group to build relationships.
Teamwork Works well with others	Works poorly with others. Has conflict with members of the team.	Works well with others, regardless of the personality.	Inspires others to collaborate together as a team and adds to organization's cohesiveness.
Technical Skill Performs job tasks well	Displays insufficient skill and knowledge for completing job tasks.	Performs all job tasks well.	Demonstrates mastery of job tasks and frequently helps others to achieve greater competence. Coaches or leads others.
Urgency Acts quickly to meet deadlines	Misses deadlines and lacks internal discipline for scheduling work appropriately.	Acts quickly and decisively to meet deadlines.	Delivers superior results before deadlines consistently. Helps others to meet commitments and organize work most effectively.

Note: The three competencies shaded in gray pertain only to department heads and front-line managers, including supervisors

Reprinted with the permission of the North Shore–Long Island Jewish Health System (rev 4/5/07)

Progressive Discipline

Progressive discipline is a process of applying escalating penalties for repeated infractions. The penalties are communicated in advance to the employee. The purpose of progressive discipline is to help an employee correct negative behavior. Termination is the ultimate result if the behavior is not corrected and there are repeated infractions accompanied by escalating penalties. Be sure you know your healthcare organization's policies and are following them.

The success of the progressive discipline process depends on the employee's willingness to exercise self-discipline in performing the job, so as not to repeat the initial offense and to avoid a more severe penalty. Progressive discipline is used to modify unacceptable behavior. It is not a punitive action.

Four Principles of Progressive Discipline

Progressive discipline is based on four principles:

- *Immediacy:* Discipline should be immediate. When possible, the employee needs to get the message that the behavior is not appropriate.

- *Known Consequences:* The employee is made aware of the consequences of his or her actions.

- *Consistency:* The employee experiences the same, consistent treatment each time a behavior is exhibited. Other employees experience the same, consistent treatment.

- *Behavior-driven:* The discipline is based on the behavior, not the person. Circumstances beyond the employee's control that cause the employee's behavior must, however, be taken into consideration (e.g., alcoholism, abuse, personal problems).

Four Steps

Progressive discipline usually is administered in a sequence of actions that grows more serious with each step. The steps—a verbal warning, written warning, suspension, and termination—are summarized in the sidebar and discussed in the paragraphs that follow. Organizations' progressive disciplinary policies differ. Check your organization's policy for progressive discipline and be sure to follow it.

Steps in Progressive Discipline

You may need to repeat a step or steps or to move ahead to the step most appropriate to a circumstance.

1. *Verbal Warning:* The employee is verbally told that the action or behavior is not acceptable.

2. *Written Warning:* A disciplinary report is completed citing the violation of policy and stating that further occurrences of the behavior will result in progressive discipline.

3. *Suspension:* If the behavior continues, the employee may be suspended without pay. The purpose of suspension is for the employee to take some time and think about the action. The employee also needs to think about how to change the behavior.

4. *Termination:* If the behavior does not change, the employee's employment relationship is terminated.

The steps you take in a particular situation depend on the circumstances of that case. In cases of just cause (i.e., theft, violence, fraud), you may move right to termination rather than go through all the steps. In other cases, repeating steps may be appropriate. Each situation requires you to act quickly once you are alerted to a situation. Each situation requires full investigation and review. Involving an objective third party is often recommended (human resources staff can be a good resource). This third party can conduct the investigation and assess the appropriateness of the discipline. Certain cases may even require you to request legal counsel. In all circumstances, you must have a witness to the progressive discipline process and appropriate documentation. Remember, if it is not documented, it did not happen.

Employee Assistance Programs

Organizations have recognized that the majority of the workforce at one time or another may face problems that interfere with daily work performance. As a supervisor, you need to know what is offered at your institution and how to access the resources. Employee assistance programs are able to address problems including but not limited to those listed in the sidebar.

> *Common Issues for Employee Assistance Programs*
> - Depression
> - Anxiety
> - Stress
> - Illness or death in the family
> - Domestic issues
> - Anger management
> - Substance abuse and other addictions
> - Elder care and child care

Use with Corrective Action
Sometimes disciplinary actions take advantage of an employee assistance program to create an opportunity for improvement. When a corrective action is indicated for an employee and you believe an employee assistance program might help, you may have the option to suggest the program as a complement to corrective action.

Employees usually are not required to participate in an employee assistance program as a condition of continued employment unless the services complement the corrective action process. Such agreements are usually separate agreements offered in conjunction with formal warnings. They must be consistent with policies and procedures regarding progressive discipline. When corrective action is in process, any referral to an employee assistance program is considered a supervisory referral. Information from supervisor referrals can be released to the employee's department only with the written consent of the employee. The information released to management and/or a supervisor is limited in scope and does not include information about the content of the confidential counseling sessions (North Shore–Long Island Jewish Health System 2006, EAP).

Conclusion

The five subjects you learned about in this chapter were employee relations, employee recognition, employee appraisals, progressive discipline, and employee assistance programs. Each of these can be said to represent the spoke on a wheel (see figure).

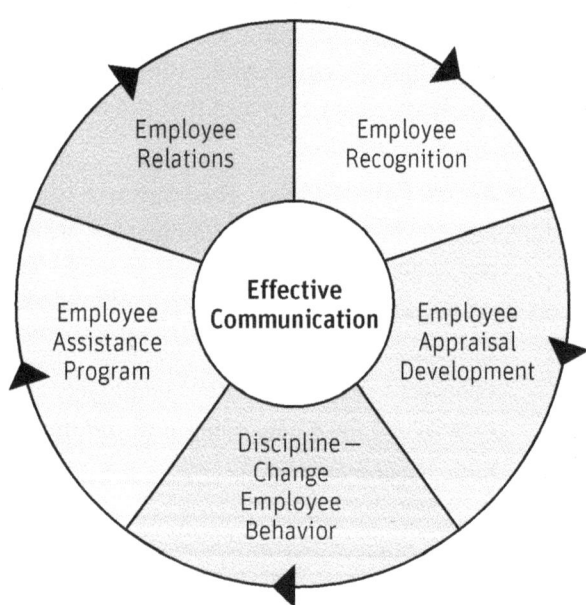

Effective communication is the hub of the wheel and the driving force for performance improvement. To move forward and advance continual improvement, all of the spokes on the wheel have to be aligned. If one spoke is out of alignment, the entire wheel will be out of alignment and opportunities for success and improvement associated with these five areas will break down.

References

Colling, R. L. 2001. *Hospital and Healthcare Security*, 4th ed. Boston: Butterworth-Heinemann, p. 155.

North Shore–Long Island Jewish Health System. "2006 Employee assistance program confidential counseling services" (part V section 3). In *Human Resources Policy and Procedures*. Lake Success, NY.

North Shore–Long Island Jewish Health System. 2006. 2006 Employee recognition program (part III section 1). In: *Human Resources Policy and Procedures*. Lake Success, NY.

The Joint Commission. 2006. HR 1.20. In: *Comprehensive Accreditation Manual for Hospitals*. Oakbrook Terrace, Ill.

The Joint Commission. 2006. HR 3.10. In: *Comprehensive Accreditation Manual for Hospitals*. Oakbrook Terrace, Ill.

The Joint Commission. 2006. HR 3.20. In: *Comprehensive Accreditation Manual for Hospitals*. Oakbrook Terrace, Ill.

Study and Review Questions

1. Which of these is one of the most important activities that management has in dealing with security employees?

    A. Tardiness

    B. Operating vehicles

    C. Communications

    D. Policy and procedures

2. Which of the following is one of the benefits of recognizing employees?

    A. Embarrasses an employee when done publicly

    B. Promotes team work and appreciation

    C. Is not cost-effective

    D. None of the above

3. Which one of the following principles is not consistent with progressive discipline?

    A. Punitive actions

    B. Immediate action

    C. Consequence of actions

    D. Consistent treatment

4. When administering progressive discipline a supervisor must do what?

    A. Always follow the four steps in sequence

    B. Can not terminate without a prior suspension

    C. Is not permitted to repeat steps

    D. Should always have a witness and document actions

Chapter 4

Authority and Control

Russell Jones, PhD, CHPA, CPP

OBJECTIVES

After studying this chapter, the student should understand the following:

- The difference between formal and informal authority
- The chain of command and the importance of empowering staff
- The control process and tools for effective management
- The three styles of authority and advantages of each
- The need for collaboration with internal departments and external agencies to establish authority and control and maintain order
- How to influence others to follow orders

Using Formal and Informal Authority

Authority levels provide the security department, or an organization, the stability and order necessary to effectively perform its functions. Authority is generally divided into two basic categories: formal and informal.

Formal Authority

When your organization gives you the power to render decisions and perform actions related to your job responsibilities, you have formal authority. Typically, your job description outlines these responsibilities and establishes the limits of the position.

Limits and responsibilities exist at every level of the organization, but vary depending on the level. For example:

- *Security officers* are usually empowered with the formal authority to challenge policy violators, patrol, respond to emergency situations, and be responsible for their actions.

- *Security supervisors* have the authority of a security officer; as well, they have the formal authority to supervise officers in daily assignments and review reports. Supervisors are responsible for themselves and the actions of the line officers under their direction.

- *Security managers* have increased formal authority. Their formal authority extends to program development, staff deployment, and accountability of the entire staff and their actions within the department.

Increases in decision making, responsibilities, and accountability continue as an individual progresses up the organizational chart. Always keep in mind that everyone is accountable to someone.

Informal Authority

Every job has gray areas of authority. Obviously, not every situation can be captured in a position description. The gray areas are referred to as the range of authority. When entrusted as a security supervisor, you are expected and need to be a leader. You must exhibit sound decision-making skills that are aligned with the philosophy of the organization. Informal authority is not granted by the organization, but developed by the individual. For example, you may have a degree of influence because you earned the respect and trust of others in the organization.

Informal authority is best developed through courtesy and respect for others. The following help establish your informal authority:

- Being knowledgeable and competent in assignments you are empowered to perform
- Projecting a positive image of the department through your interactions with customers

Generally, persons with informal authority are team players, and individuals displaying these characteristics may eventually become leaders. Not surprisingly, individuals with significant informal authority generally have a higher potential for career advancement.

Understanding Chain of Command

The chain of command is often described as an unbroken line of authority. As a security supervisor, you are within that chain of command. You are responsible for knowing the answer to each of these questions:

- Who do I go to?
- Who am I responsible for?

To ensure authority and control are maintained, you must understand the need for a chain of command and its impact on maintaining order. Authority has been described as the "rights inherent in a managerial position to give orders and expect these orders to be obeyed" (Robbins 2000). The command you are given allows you to preserve the entire chain of command (see graphic for the typical structure). The communication you are expected to provide to those above and below you is what makes the chain of command a necessity to the organization. To ensure the chain of command is being met, you must plan and take corrective actions. What you measure is more critical than how you measure.

The concepts of chain of command, authority, and unity of command have substantially less relevance today because of advances in computer technology and trends toward empowering employees (Robbins 2000). The next section explains how empowerment works.

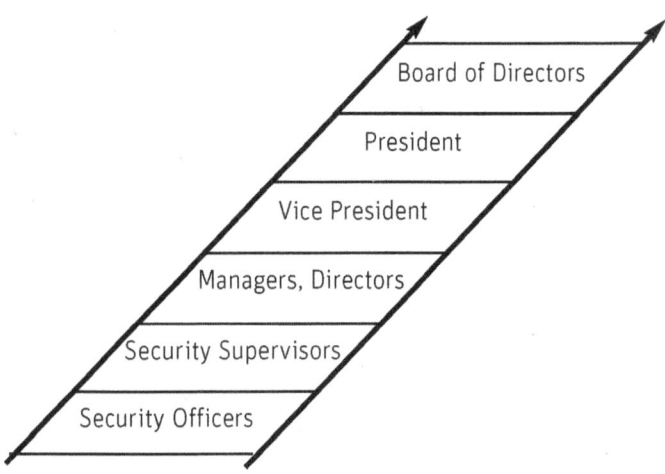

Using the Empowerment Model

Organizations are moving away from rigid management authority and toward open decision making. Here are three reasons why:

- Lower-level employees today can access information in seconds that, 20 years ago, was available only to top managers.
- Computer technology increasingly allows employees anywhere in an organization to communicate with anyone else without going through formal channels.
- The concepts of authority and maintaining the chain of command are increasingly less relevant as operating employees are being empowered to make decisions that previously were reserved for management (Robbins 2000).

Do not let the rigidity of formal organizational charts hinder successes in open decision making. Instead, recognize that communication between different levels is more important than ever.

Your good judgment is also essential. Good judgment enables you to make the best decisions possible. You are responsible for your decisions and any decisions that affect the accountability of the entire management team.

Supervisors who exhibit delegation, team development, and self-management skills are the most successful. If the entire security team replicates the thoughts and actions of such a supervisor, the supervisor would ensure not only outstanding personal success, but also greater success for department personnel.

Understanding the Process of Control

The span of control separates employees into levels. Each level usually has a specific number of employees and a leader. Using the span of control, organizations can improve their effectiveness.

The span of control is invaluable to a supervisor. Decisions are best made by those closest to the action. Line staff and/or the supervisor have more details and knowledge about ongoing security problems and incidents than do top managers.

A supervisor needs to be a critical thinker. You need to maintain control of your level and support all other levels as needed. You must, for example, give support to the people who delegated control of your level to you. To control most unpredictable incidents, you need these abilities:

- Ability to influence subordinates
- Ability to guide a behavior
- Ability to render imperative decisions

Even when you have these abilities, a situation can break down if you take on more authority and control than you have been given. You must consider the impact on other areas of the institution, such as patient care or other clinical functions. One example would be visitors who appear angry and emotional over the care of their loved one. Clinical staff may want them removed. Certainly, control needs to be maintained, but the decision should involve other clinical or administrative staff. Doing so ensures the result is best for all involved. You want to ensure that any action taken is not performed in a manner that could jeopardize the organization's mission.

Tools for Effective Management

To effectively manage staff (officers, agents, investigators, or whatever title your employees are known by), the security supervisor counts on several tools (Robbins 2000, p. 57):

- The authority needed to discipline
- Input on who is assigned to the unit
- A voice when staff are considered for promotion
- The authority to require additional training
- The authority to communicate to your own staff, including sending instructions, memos, and so on
- The freedom to measure your staff's performance without interference

Performance is the ultimate goal of supervisors (Sennewald 2003, p. 62). The only way to receive respect and obtain trust from your subordinates is to use your own judgment and accept the need to make final decisions.

Unity of Command

Violations of the principle of unity of command are not usually due to the design of the organization. These occur more by accident than design. Sennewald, for example, points out that special events and non-routine occasions tend to bring out more executives than usual (Sennewald 2003, p. 17). The best way to ensure unity of command is to educate everyone on how security supervisors can help with the overall activities of the organization.

Training

Training must be continuous for supervisors. New supervisors are often quick to discover that they are ill-prepared for their new responsibilities. They are sensitive to their deficiencies and lack confidence in handling problems and people.

Subordinates are very quick to sense this absence of confidence. Some will not be at all sympathetic. Rather, they will capitalize on the apparent weakness to their own advantage, especially those who jealously believe they should have received that promotion.

Becoming a Change Agent

Businesses rarely succeed with sustainable transformation initiatives unless they are led from the top. This holds true as security programs change, too. The individual in charge of the security department needs to embrace this concept and be willing to accept and adapt to change. Even if the change is small, you can create your own model within the organization to create a positive outcome.

Understanding the scope of the task at hand and creating a model to measure the effectiveness of the change are key. Creating a benchmark tool such as a survey will allow any manager to change effectively without wasting energy and time.

Applying Appropriate Styles of Authority

Several styles of management are used in the direction of personnel. Which do you use? Which should you use? Motivating subordinates to be productive members of the organization is your goal. Consider the three types—authoritarian, laissez-faire, and quality management—and what adjustments you may need to make on the whole and in specific situations.

There is no right or wrong method to apply across the board. Rather, to be effective in certain situations, you must employ the appropriate style of authority. Your decision on which style to use may differ depending on the situation or individuals involved.

Authoritarian

In the authoritarian style, you, as the supervisor, see yourself in total charge and are the enforcer in the department. You expect all subordinates to do as you order, without question.

Be mindful of the disadvantages of the authoritarian supervisory style. Being overly authoritarian can lead to the following:

- *Creation of a Tense Work Environment:* Because explanations are not provided, subordinates have many questions as to why things are done in a certain way.
- *Attitude of "There's No Room for Participatory Democracy in Business":* General sense is that decisions have to be made quickly, that there is no time to consult everybody, and, besides, too may independent thinkers usually spoil a decision.
- *Feelings of Hostility and Aggression:* Subordinates may harbor negative feelings against the supervisor.
- *Limitation of Employees' Freedom of Thought or Empowerment:* Subordinates feel they are not allowed to make decisions.
- *Over-reliance on Supervisor:* Subordinates fail to accomplish assignments in the supervisor's absence.

Laissez-faire

The laissez-faire style of management is a less structured, hands-off approach to supervision. Under laissez-faire management, employees are left to do as they please—including setting their own goals, making their own policies, and following their own procedures. A laissez-faire supervisor believes that workers do their best when left alone to provide self-direction and self-motivation.

As with the authoritarian style, you need to be aware of the disadvantages of laissez-faire style supervision:

- *Reduced Productivity and Decreased Quality of Service:* Supervisor may be required to complete assignments avoided by staff.
- *Risk of Misperception About Supervisor's Level of Interest:* Subordinates may assume supervisors do not care about employees' work or the performance of subordinates.

Quality Management

Authoritarian and laissez-faire styles of supervision can be seen as the two extremes. Blending the two is referred to as the quality management style. Quality management—a group-oriented management style—is the preferred supervisory style.

Historically in the security profession, the tendency has been to use the authoritarian style, but a shift is occurring. The trend is to use the skills and abilities of your individual officers in a group-oriented management style. Group-oriented management gives employees the ability to make decisions that positively impact their daily assignments. This style of supervision looks like this:

- Communication is open
- Explanations are given and reasons are provided for policies and procedures
- Employees have increased pride in their work and a sense of ownership
- Eventually, productivity increases and the quality of work is higher

Work teams are one technique of quality management. Work teams involve all members of the department. Members are given clear parameters and performance measures for the team. Since security officers have day-to-day contact with customers while performing their assignments, the officers become empowered to determine the best method to meet their customers' needs. The supervisor becomes a coach, trainer, and source of feedback, rather than a disciplinarian.

Through a supervisor's monitoring and influence, productivity and pride in workmanship are increased. Members of the department work toward meeting their target goals. Unmet goals require intervention—through performance reviews. Employees also work with each other to resolve difficulties. The downside of this style is that employees must want to participate and make a difference. Lack of participation can lead to a laissez-faire environment.

Open, two-way communication is vital for success with quality management. You must be conscious of your style of management and recognize when to use a specific style. In some situations, the authoritarian style must be used.

Emergency Response. Emergency situations call for authoritarian supervision at the time of the event. In the planning phases, though, the quality management style brings benefits. In an emergency response, decisions must be made quickly. There is little time for discussion and input. People understand that. In planning responses to emergency situations, though, the quality management style is of value. Encourage security officers to be involved in planning. During that time, they can voice opinions and concerns. After an incident is over, again seek officer input to reveal ways to improve. In this way, when an incident occurs, the plan is quickly and effectively executed by the department and supported by the organization.

Matching Styles to Employees and Situations. What makes the choice of supervisory style difficult is the fact that different individuals respond better under different situations. Recognize which method works best in each situation, and use imagination and creativity to address individual circumstances, individual officers, and situations. The officer will show you whether an authoritarian approach or laissez-faire approach is needed. If uncertain, or you encounter extreme difficulties after you have attempted to resolve the issue, use the chain of command and discuss the issue with your supervisor.

A vital consideration in your overall effectiveness is the degree to which you earn the respect of the security officers. In this regard, supervision by example can play a key role. For example, you may hear a security officer saying, "I am not a real fan of Supervisor Smith, but I'll say one thing about her: she'd never ask me to do something she wouldn't do herself."

Using an Inverted Chain of Command

In many organizations, managers allow their staff to safely "fail." The inverted chain of command encourages supervisors to place themselves in the front-line employees' shoes. This enables front-line staff to be at the top of the authority chain and the supervisor at the bottom. With this model, staff feel empowered to accept change, accept responsibility, and be encouraged to take ownership of the opportunity. For example, an officer can be put on one of the hospital's committees or be given responsibility for running the lost and found.

Collaborating with Internal Departments

In recent years, it has become clear that security supervisors cannot work alone to provide a safe, secure environment. The officers and the authority and control given to all of us must be accepted, respected, and acknowledged by other departments to arrive at success. In the healthcare industry, patients, visitors, and staff need to rely on our direction and knowledge to understand the goals and missions of the institutions. The standards of care are no longer only decided by clinical decision makers. The nursing, medical, facilities, risk management, legal, and other quality assurance departments need to understand the capability of the security officers and the resources they have been given to create a safe and secure environment. Non-clinical staff, such as security and other ancillary services, are essential. They respond to routine calls for prompt service as well as the more difficult situations that may result in declaring disaster phases.

As a security supervisor, you can control the scene by using the authority given to you in ways that appropriately engage and empower others. Getting others involved, in an orderly fashion, allows you to accomplish many tasks at once. You can ensure the level of care and lessen anxiety at the same time—this is usually not an easy task. Keep in mind that your subordinates may be asked to perform tasks that are not commonly required by them. As the leader assigned to coordinate with other departments, you must provide confidence to other departments that your authority and control is evident and necessary. The relationship between security and others should present no difficulties. The interface and collaborating efforts should solve potentially disruptive incidents shared by both departments. Therefore, the goals are met by eliminating conflicts that may arise if collaboration does not occur.

Collaborating with External Departments

As a security supervisor, you must understand that at any time you may need and rely on external support from local, state, and federal authorities. When this occurs, your level of authority should not be compromised; however, your level of control may be shared—if it is not removed due to the nature of the incident you have been called to control. The collaborative efforts of these agencies are necessary; however, your facility may not be familiar to them. You will be asked to facilitate quick access to the scene without compromising patient care or creating pandemonium in other areas of the institution.

You make these collaborations successful by being proactive. Meet with agencies before any need arises. A working relationship and continued sharing of response plans ensures the type of response you may need. These ongoing meetings also grow a professional relationship. Both internal and external agencies need this. Establishing these relationships opens communication lines. Thus, suggestions and ongoing recommendations can be shared easily. The interaction and support can provide an extra measure of safety to the institution.

Maintaining an Orderly Facility

Beyond the supervisory responsibility to manage security personnel, you also are responsible for maintaining an orderly facility. A few of the expectations of security personnel are highlighted below:

- Interact with other departments
- Promote organizational philosophies
- Perform the daily functions entrusted to the security department—e.g., deterring criminal activities, being available for service requests, creating a safe work environment

As the supervisor, you are the channel of communication between departments. You ensure that the mission is accomplished. You can accomplish this through a positive attitude, empathy, dedication, and positive rapport.

Influencing Others to Follow Orders

Paramount to the security supervisor's and security program's success is the need to get others to follow orders. The security program should be clearly understood by the supervisors outlining the requests and expectations from the organization.

Security orders are generally in two forms: long-standing orders (such as policies and procedures) and specific orders (those unique to a given situation, such as a temporary change in the building lockdown schedule). To have orders followed, you, and thus your department, must be able to provide a degree of motivation or influence. There are a variety of theories on how to influence employees to follow directions. Five recommendations are given in the sidebar.

Influencing Others to Follow Orders

- Motivate subordinates to follow orders by setting a good example in following orders yourself.

- Make certain that orders are clear, concise, and understood. Be aware that what to do may be understood, but how to do it may not.

- Be thoroughly familiar with the levels and experience of subordinates. Delegate assignments to those officers whose experience is sufficient to assume the assignment. Focus on coaching those individuals who are unfamiliar with assignments to increase productivity and knowledge.

- Conduct yourself in a professional manner that influences loyalty in others; in return, you develop subordinates' confidence so they follow orders.

- Explain why assignments or orders are to be done. In doing so, you can make the assignment more meaningful. In the long run, the explanation may increase productivity and clarify the importance of organizational and departmental goals. This may not apply in every situation, but can be a useful tool.

Supervisors are valued by their ability to get others to follow orders. Promotions, pay increases, bonuses, and all the prizes of management rest on your ability to get assignments accomplished through others.

Conclusion

The success of any security program resides with effective management by supervisory personnel. Your organization must recognize formal and informal authority and realize that limits to authority exist. When you reach those limits, use the chain of command. Remain firm but fair in your management and disciplinary styles. As a supervisor, you must be able to predict and manage change, but, most importantly, you must remain flexible. Being able to empower subordinates and work with other agencies, internal or external, is essential to a supervisor's success. Always be professional by maintaining self-control and leading by example.

References

Robbins, S. P. 2000. *Managing Today.* Upper Saddle River, NJ: Prentice Hall, Inc., pp. 241–242.

Sennewald, C. A. 2003. *Effective Security Management.* Boston: Butterworth-Heinemann, pp. 57, 17, 62.

Bibliography

Colling, R. L. 2001. *Hospital and Healthcare Security*, 4th ed. Boston: Butterworth-Heinemann.

Green, G. and R. J. Fischer. 1998. *Introduction to Security*, 6th ed. Boston: Butterworth-Heinemann.

Robbins, S. P. 2000. *Managing Today*, 2nd ed. Upper Saddle River, NJ: Prentice Hall Inc.

Sennewald, C. A. 2003. *Effective Security Management*, 4th ed. Boston: Butterworth-Heinemann.

Study and Review Questions

1. Which of the following describes the two basic categories of authority?

    A. Formal and official

    B. Formal and informal

    C. Informal and management

    D. Informal and official

2. The chain of command is often described by which term?

    A. Line of authority

    B. Chain of order

    C. Unbroken line of authority

    D. Unity of command

3. The security profession has a tendency toward which style of management?

    A. Authoritarian

    B. Laissez-faire

    C. Quality

    D. Superior

4. Which of the following is not a trait of a successful supervisor?

    A. Delegation

    B. Team development

    C. Self-managing skills

    D. Span of control

Chapter 5

Leadership

Anjanette Hebert, CHPA

OBJECTIVES

After studying this chapter, the student should understand the following:

- Effective qualities of successful leaders
- The difference between managers and leaders
- Strategies leaders use to get results
- How to identify effective leadership styles and delegation of authority—and how and when to use these appropriately
- The principle of leadership by example

There is power in thinking big, and thinking big requires risk taking. Great leaders are risk takers. They have courage to believe in their own vision and to lead and, probably most importantly, the courage to give colleagues and subordinates authority and power.

Healthcare facilities accredited through The Joint Commission are familiar with the following definition of leadership: leadership is a process consisting of planning, directing, integrating, and improving performance. This is a broad and simplistic definition for a complex process. On a more personal level, leadership is a function of knowing oneself, having a vision that is well communicated, building trust among colleagues, and taking effective action to realize your own leadership potential. Becoming a successful leader without taking a few risks is unlikely.

To live up to this definition of leadership while working in the healthcare environment, you must create and participate in the vision and future of the institution. Leading effectively in an environment in which you do not support the vision is difficult. If communicating the vision and building trust are elements of leadership, only an inspired leader can truly direct the day-to-day activities leading to successful fulfillment of the mission.

One of the essential attributes of a successful leader is enough self-confidence to be able to admit your mistakes, recognize what went wrong as early as possible and then set about rectifying the situation. The qualities and characteristics identified in this chapter reveal how leaders use the learned traits and skills of effective leadership to establish expectations, plans, and priorities so that their staffs can continuously improve their performance to meet the needs of the healthcare organization's mission, vision, and values.

Management Style Versus Leadership

What is the difference between management style and leadership? In their book *Leaders*, Warren Bennis and Burt Nanus made this distinction between managers and leaders: Managers do things right while leaders do the right thing. Some notable differences are these:

- *Managers* manage the status quo; they oversee a department or process to ensure efficiency and productivity. *Leaders,* on the other hand, go beyond that to create organizational change.
- *Managers* maintain the balance of the operation, while *leaders* create new approaches and imagine new areas to explore.
- Where *managers* act to limit choices by holding staff accountable to established procedures and processes, *leaders* work to inspire staff to challenge the established procedures and process and to develop fresh approaches to long-standing problems. This often involves taking risks that would not be possible without the leader's courage to believe in his or her vision and giving subordinates authority and power.

The essence of leadership is found in the leader's ability to move the department to a higher level of performance. Bennis and Nanus provide a clear definition of leadership: "Leadership is what gives an organization its vision and its ability to translate the vision into reality."

Characteristics of Good Leadership

Successful leaders have profound effects on their employees and must realize how their position and authority influences the staff. Dwight D. Eisenhower once said, "Leadership is the art of getting someone else to do what you want done because he or she wants to do it." That kind of influence has much longer lasting effects than getting someone to do something through fear or intimidation. Good leadership displays the characteristics listed below. Each is discussed separately in the paragraphs that follow:

- Has a hands-off management style
- Focuses on staff retention and morale
- Champions the staff
- Emphasizes accountability

Style

One challenge that plagues many potential leaders is the tendency to micro-manage others. Micro-managing can stifle creativity and spontaneity, ultimately impeding growth and leading to dissatisfaction and low morale among staff. A good leader recognizes when to get out of the way to let people do their jobs and when to challenge them. George S. Patton once said, "Never tell people how to do things. Tell them what to do, and they will surprise you with their ingenuity." A leader who never challenges staff members' belief that they can not achieve beyond a certain level limits the success of the entire program.

Staff Retention and Morale

Staff retention and morale are areas where the leader has profound influence. In today's society, employees are not loyal to organizations, they are loyal to people. Studies have proven that when workers are paid at fair market value, they are more likely to rank feeling appreciated as more important than higher wages or even job security.

Championing

Pride building, instilling self-esteem in staff, and building support for the organization are rare leadership qualities that have been touted for as long as literature on leadership has been available. In times of plunging profits, pride building is especially difficult. In such difficult times, truly inspirational leaders emerge. Not uncommonly, however, a leader who champions staff appreciation may be thought of as "warm and fuzzy." Nothing could be further from the truth! A great leader recognizes that work is personal and what happens to someone at work is taken personally.

The most effective leaders know that the best work is inspired not by economics alone, but also by emotions. The best work is done in a balanced environment. Leaders engage employees as allies, creating a sense of accomplishment, camaraderie, and emotional attachment. This helps achieve big goals because employees are inspired to take risks along with their leader. Such leaders believe that personalizing the workplace fosters a commitment and loyalty that could not otherwise be attained.

Accountability

At the same time, effectiveness requires that the leader hold himself or herself and others accountable. While employees need to feel rewarded and appreciated for a job well done, they also must see discipline imposed for unacceptable work or behavior. Reward without accountability is meaningless.

Without effective leadership, a staff rises only to a level of expectation that maintains the status quo or to a level of marginal performance. Employees who are managed rather than led do not venture beyond basic expectations. Managed staffs usually do not take risks to seek a higher level of performance. Managed staffs usually meet the minimum requirements to get by.

Basic Functions of Effective Leadership

William D. Hitt in *The Leader-Manager* identified eight actions of a successful leader. A successful leader develops the team, creates vision, clarifies values, positions the staff, communicates effectively, empowers staff, coaches staff, and measures success. These eight functions are described more fully in the sidebar.

> *Actions of a Successful Leader*
> - ***Develops the Team:*** Develops a team of highly qualified officers who are jointly responsible for achieving the department's goals.
> - ***Creates the Vision:*** Constructs a crystal-clear mental picture of what the staff should become and then transmits this vision to others.
> - ***Clarifies the Values:*** Identifies the organizational values and communicates these values through words and actions.
> - ***Positions:*** Develops an effective strategy for moving the group from its present position toward the vision.
> - ***Communicates:*** Achieves a common understanding with others by using all modes of communications effectively.
> - ***Empowers:*** Motivates others by raising them to their "better selves."
> - ***Coaches:*** Helps staff members develop the skills they need to achieve excellence.
> - ***Measures:*** Identifies the critical success factors associated with the group's operation and gauges progress on the basis of these factors.
>
> Source: Hitt, W. D. 1988. The Leader-Manager: Guidelines for Action. Columbus, Ohio: Battelle Press.

As a supervisor, you can apply these eight actions to contribute to your own leadership effectiveness. A security supervisor who takes these actions is very likely to be an effective leader.

Types of Leaders

A leader's style is defined as the way he or she focuses his or her attention and interacts with staff. The leader sets the tone for subordinates and communicates expectations. Not every leader has the same style. Leadership theory provides a means to understand more about the relationship of leadership to effectiveness. Burns (1978) identified two types of leadership: transformational and transactional.

The Transformational Leader

Transformational leadership (formally known as charismatic leadership) has the characteristics of motivating others by using visionary, inspirational, and intellectually stimulating approaches and paying high attention to the individual differences among people. Transformational leaders assume that people will follow a person who inspires them, that a person with vision and passion can achieve great things, and that the way to get things done is by injecting enthusiasm and energy in people. A transformational leader goes beyond his or her self-interest for the good of the organization or group.

Moral Leadership Style. One of the traits that help transformational leaders achieve effectiveness in their role as supervisor is a moral leadership style. The moral leadership style demonstrates how effective that individual is as a person and how well they are understood by others. The importance of your behavior in influencing the ethical conduct of your staff cannot be understated. What the leader does as a person affects the staff.

As a security supervisor, your honesty and credibility have to remain unimpeachable. The staff wants to follow a moral leader. Your organization can give you the power to lead, your knowledge can give you the ability to lead, but only demonstrated character and courage in difficult situations earn you the right to lead in the eyes of your subordinates.

Earning Respect and Support. Respect and support from the staff are earned and cannot be demanded based on a position title. Subordinates who respect their leaders emulate the leader's style and actions. Effective leaders set examples and discipline themselves to achieve and exceed the standards established for themselves and staff. If the leader fails to surpass staff expectations or the standards to which the staff are evaluated, then the leader's credibility is questioned and departmental effectiveness declines. The leader's own effectiveness depends largely on whether or not the leader has the willing support and respect of subordinates.

To earn the respect and support of your staff, make the following your guiding principles:

- Never openly criticize management or say derogatory things about others
- Never question organizational policy and procedures with your subordinates
- Always exceed the standards established for your staff
- Be eager to share credit and render praise with staff
- Avoid disciplining staff for errors or mistakes similar to those you have committed

The Transactional Leader

Transactional leaders, in contrast, assume that people are motivated by reward and punishment; that social systems work best with a clear chain of command; that when people have agreed to do a job they cede all authority to their manager as part of the deal; and that the prime purpose of a subordinate is to do what the manager assigns. Transactional leadership has the characteristics of defining contracts and identifying mistakes in others.

Bureaucratic Leadership Style. Transactional leaders believe authority is derived from governing rules or policies. Managerial functions should be carried out according to calculable rules without regard for persons. The primary function of this type of leader is to communicate and enforce rules. Transactional leaders believe employees should be appointed on the basis of their technical skills and staff should be subject to strict and systematic discipline and control. The work of the leader is that of planning, organizing, staffing, staff development, communicating, motivating, and measuring.

Progressive Leadership Style. Transactional leaders with a progressive leadership style set objectives and then go about reaching them in an organized, orderly, and conscious way. This leader's role in the organization is to achieve organizational objectives through effective and efficient deployment of departmental, physical, and fiscal resources. Progressive leaders are educated, trained, and skilled in effective leadership principles, methods, and skills.

The Essentials of Effective Leadership

Leaders should always endeavor to train their staffs to become good leaders. Note this key difference between effective leaders and insecure managers: Effective leaders try to develop the power within their subordinates whenever they can and then gather all this power and use it as the energizing force to accomplish even greater goals and tasks. Insecure managers, in contrast, often try to suppress the leadership of subordinates because they fear it may rival their own. With this distinction in mind, here are some essentials to effective leadership.

Effective leaders...
- Work systematically at managing their time and are not afraid to delegate
- Focus on outward contributions
- Build on the strengths of individuals
- Motivate others to levels of superior performance to produce outstanding results
- Make effective decisions
- Have infectious optimism
- Are team builders

Based on extensive research on leadership, staffs of effective leaders...
- Emulate the leader
- Strive to meet the leader's expectations
- Want to do more than they are expected to do, are willing to take risks
- Want to achieve a higher level of performance
- Demonstrate a higher degree of innovation
- Will extend themselves toward personal and professional development

Delegation: A Leadership Tool

An effective leader needs to manage time effectively and feel comfortable sharing power and authority with staff. By delegating, leaders multiply their effectiveness through others. Delegation is a way of assigning to others part or all of a job to free time for other important issues. Delegation builds skills and morale among staff, but challenges staff members to try new things. As a supervisor, you can delegate the authority to accomplish a task, but the responsibility for successful completion remains with you. When you are delegating, you need to delegate to staff members who have the skills to successfully complete the task.

Benefits for the Supervisor

As a leader you can benefit by delegating authority to others. The benefits include the following:
- Helps you accomplish more through others
- Frees you to devote time to the most pressing matters as well as long-term planning
- Helps you grow in the role as coach to your subordinates
- Gives you a source of new ideas
- Increases your capacity to meet deadlines

Benefits for Staff

Subordinates and staff benefit from delegation in the following ways:
- Gives staff a better understanding of your job as supervisor
- Promotes more of a transforming (as opposed to bureaucratic) relationship between you and the staff
- Allows staff to assume greater responsibilities in their job roles
- Provides staff with professional growth opportunities on the job

Delegation is not a gimmick used by a leader to get rid of work. Rather, delegation is a leadership strategy to get better resources committed to accomplishing work. Effective delegation is the result of serious planning. You must clearly understand what is involved before the delegation takes place and then follow through with your plan for delegation.

Self-assessment of Leadership Skills

To evaluate your own leadership skills, conduct the self-assessment on this page.

Assess Your Leadership Skills

Rate yourself on a scale from 0 to 5 regarding each of the following questions.

    5 = to a great extent
    4 = to a large extent
    3 = to a moderate extent
    2 = to a slight extent
    1 = very little
    0 = not at all

1. Do I accept and enjoy the role of a leader? ____
2. Am I action oriented and do I have a strong drive to accomplish and achieve? ____
3. Am I willing "to stand up and be counted"— even with an unpopular view? ____
4. Am I able to abandon outmoded assumptions and experiment with alternative concepts? ____
5. Do I have the necessary power to empower staff and resources to implement an idea? ____
6. Do I consistently treat staff fairly? ____
7. Do I demonstrate the ability to set direction for the department beyond the daily routine? ____
8. Am I able to obtain acceptance of the department vision by all team members? ____
9. Do I support the department vision as well as the goals of the healthcare organization? ____
10. Do I create an environment that fosters trust among the staff? ____
11. Am I successful in translating the organization's values into a reality that is manifest in the staff's daily behavior? ____
12. Do I show true concern for each staff member as a person? ____
13. Do I motivate others by enthusiasm and optimism? ____
14. Do I have the ability to bring out the best in subordinates? ____
15. Am I able to make staff members feel that they are winners? ____
16. Do I take a personal interest in the career development of each department member? ____
17. Am I effective in developing subordinates to become leaders? ____
18. Am I an effective delegator? ____
19. Am I actively developing one or more backups for my position? ____
20. Do I provide recognition for superior performance? ____

                                                                    Total score: ____

Where do you stand?

86–100	Strong leadership skills and qualities
70–85	Moderate leadership skills and qualities
50–69	Slight leadership abilities
0–49	Need to develop basic leadership abilities and qualities

Conclusion

In his book *The Right to Lead*, John C. Maxwell states, "Your talk talks and your walk talks, but your walk talks louder than your talk talks." In other words, what you do influences staff much more than what you say. As a supervisor, how you conduct yourself can determine the success of your department and your ability to motivate others to share in the vision for the department and the organization.

Effective leadership skills are not necessarily second nature. Rather, as a supervisor, you must learn them and put them into practice. Wanting to be a leader and believing that you can lead are only the starting points on the path to effective leadership. Mastering the art of leadership comes with mastery of the self. Ultimately, leadership development is a process of self-development.

Bibliography

Accreditation Manual for Hospitals (Leadership Standards). 2007. Oakbrook Terrace, Ill: The Joint Commission.

Aspen Reference Group. 1995. *Safety and Security Administration in Health Care Facilities*. Gaithersburg, Md: Aspen Publishers Inc.

Bass, B. M., B. J. Avolio and L. Atwater. 1996. The transformational and transactional leadership of men and women. *Applied Psychology: An International Review* 45:5–34.

Bennis, W. 1989. *On Becoming a Leader*. New York: Addison Wesley.

Burns, J. M. 1978. *Leadership*. New York: Harper & Row.

Byrne, J. A. 2003 Aug. How to lead: getting extraordinary performance when you can't pay for it. *Fast Company*, p. 62.

Cook, T. M. and R. A. Russell. 1980. *Contemporary Operations Management*. Englewood Cliffs, NJ: Prentice-Hall Inc.

Downey, E. 2005. "The relationship of transformational leadership to organizational performance of hospital-based disaster coordinators using the multi-factor leadership questionnaire." PhD diss., Tulane University School of Public Health and Tropical Medicine, New Orleans.

Galle, W. P. and D. A. Level. 1980. *Business Communication: Theory and Practice*. Dallas: Business Publication Inc.

Hitt, W. D. 1990. *Ethics and Leadership: Putting Theory into Practice*. Columbus, Ohio: Battelle Press.

Hitt, W. D. 1988. *The Leader-Manager: Guidelines for Action*. Columbus, Ohio: Battelle Press.

Hitt, W. D. 1992. *Thoughts on Leadership*. Columbus, Ohio: Battelle Press.

Lauer, C. S. 11 Aug 2003. Leading the way: managers are important, but leaders really make things happen (publisher's letter) (leadership in the healthcare industry) (column). *Modern Healthcare* 33(32):30.

Maxwell, J. C. 2001. *The Right To Lead*. Nashville: J. Countryman.

Novak, W. 1984. *Iacocca: an Autobiography*. Toronto: Bantam Books.

Ramsey, R. D. Sep 2003. The power of thinking big. *Supervision* 64(9):8–9.

Yammarino, F. J. and B. M. Bass. 1990. "Long-term forecasting of transformational leadership and its effects among naval officers: some preliminary findings." In: *Measures of Leadership*. Clark K. E. and M. B. Clark (eds.). West Orange, NY: Leadership Library of America, pp. 151–169.

Study and Review Questions

1. What is the difference between managers and leaders?

    A. Leaders do the right thing

    B. Managers do the right thing

    C. Leaders do things right

    D. None of the above

2. According to this chapter, how many basic functions are there of effective leadership?

    A. Six

    B. Nine

    C. Eight

    D. Twelve

3. Which type of leader motivates others by using inspirational approaches?

    A. Transactional leader

    B. Transformational leader

    C. Departmental leader

    D. Bureaucratic leader

4. Which of the following best defines delegation as described in this chapter?

    A. A way of getting things done

    B. A way of not doing things yourself

    C. A way of trying to make the department look good

    D. A way to multiply effectiveness through others

Chapter 6

Handling Complaints and Grievances

Paul Mains, CPP

OBJECTIVES

After studying this chapter, the student should understand the following:

- Stress factors involved in healthcare
- How dissatisfaction manifests itself
- Proactive supervisory techniques that help prevent complaints
- The results of dissatisfaction
- Problem-solving strategies for supervisors

As a supervisor, you are a fixer. Fixing personnel matters that keep the department from running smoothly is part of your job. Maintaining peace, harmony, and productivity is a basic element of supervisory responsibility. You cannot achieve this if your employees are consistently unhappy. Other chapters in this manual address morale; this chapter looks at how to prevent complaints from developing and how to handle formal complaints and grievances an employee may have about the workplace.

Complaints that are not addressed fester like wounds. You must treat the person with the problem or the department will become infected. An infected workforce is not productive. Ignoring a problem does not make it go away; rather, ignoring a problem allows it to get worse.

As you seek to resolve complaints and to prevent them from occurring in the first place, recognize that you are in the middle in these situations. You represent the security management to the security officers and the security officers to the security management. Your goal is to maintain a quality work product while harmonizing both the officers and management.

Complaints and Grievances

A complaint is a statement of unhappiness. A grievance is a complaint about a process. Both need attention and may require action. Management often believes that the best person to hear and resolve complaints and grievances is the first-line supervisor.

The Supervisor's Role

You must actively engage in this process rather than shy away from it. Mastering the ability to problem-solve complaints and grievances builds trust and loyalty among your subordinates. This skill serves you well on the road to career development.

You must bring knowledge, ability, and communication skills to succeed in this effort. You need a solid foundation upon which to build your response. A written policy for handling complaints and grievances is critical to this process. You need to thoroughly understand applicable policies and be able to interpret them; this is fundamental. Know what you are talking about. Bluffing is not an option.

There is a direct relationship between turnover and the goals of job satisfaction and promotion. Knowing what creates or aggravates employee concerns helps you plan to avoid problems and, if necessary, deal with them at an early stage. To be effective, you must become adept at this process. Helping resolve employee complaints and grievances is part of the job. Be aware also that your advancement may depend on your skills in this area. Some basic skills are necessary:

- *The ability to communicate* is primary.
- *The ability to pay attention* to what is going on around you will keep little problems from becoming big problems.
- *The ability to care* about things and particularly about people shows through and will make or break you in terms of problem solving. If people think you do not care, they will not trust you. If they do not trust you, they will not trust the administration. This line of thinking can lead employees to rationalization, which leads to poor performance.

Stress Factors

One of the keys to job satisfaction in healthcare settings is the desire to help people, especially people in trouble. Typically, people working in this field are drawn to this type of helping environment. Working in the healthcare environment can be very rewarding, but the work has its share of stressful situations. Ideally, your new employees are aware of many of these stressors before coming to the job. Unfortunately, this is often not the case. Coaching new employees early in their tenure mitigates some of these stressors. The following are common stressors that can affect your employees:

- Shift work
- Long hours with repetitious job tasks
- Odd or split days off
- Schedule changes due to emergency conditions
- Victim and patient trauma
- Dealing with angry, upset, grieving patients and family
- Co-worker issues

Sources of Employee Dissatisfaction

Today's officers want more input. As a supervisor, you must listen and act as an agent of change. Given this work's inherent stressors (described in the list above), employee dissatisfaction can manifest itself in the following ways:

- Unhappiness with the inability to adjust shifts
- Perception of management not listening to or acting on concerns
- Concern with professional growth within the organization
- Perception that discipline is inconsistently applied
- Inability to get along with or disrespect for certain co-workers
- Boredom brought on by the perceived lack of job challenge
- Outside concerns that may not be known to employer

The Supervisor's Proactive Steps

Effective supervisors are proactive. Pay attention to what is going on in the workplace. Address each source of dissatisfaction mentioned above and others you know of to minimize and reduce opportunities for dissatisfaction. Review the sidebar for positive steps that can reduce negative opportunities.

Chapter 6: Handling Complaints and Grievances

Addressing Potential Sources of Employee Dissatisfaction Through Proactive Supervision

- Have a clear job description containing job expectations and responsibilities that are specific, realistic, and obtainable
- Provide adequate training and retraining on an ongoing basis
- Maintain and replace as necessary supplied equipment
- Provide a forum for employee feedback
- Provide a lead officer, supervisor, or person to report to on each shift
- Have a clean, safe environment in which to do the job
- Establish and maintain an employee recognition program
- Ensure officers know about and have access to the employee assistance program
- Create an information distribution chain that documents that officers have received policy and procedural changes
- Treat all employees fairly
- Maintain consistent disciplinary procedures
- Have a realistic career development plan
- Have flexibility built in to accommodate special situations such as childcare, transportation, and spouse issues

Proactively address as many of the potential sources of employee dissatisfaction as possible. Use the employee handbook and existing policy. The employee handbook should be updated yearly and policy revisited on a regular, documented basis. Using these two resources, you can find most of the significant areas of expected or prohibited behavior.

Results of Dissatisfaction

Unhappy employees manifest their dissatisfaction in a number of ways. Be alert to these:

- Attitude changes
- Excessive sick time
- Performance declines
- Tardiness
- Work quality issues
- Late or incomplete work
- Carelessness
- Safety violations
- Hygiene and appearance changes
- Co-worker issues
- Personality changes

Some changes are easily noticed, while others are not. Remember that unless you address the problem, you are allowing it to get worse.

Intervention

If you pay attention, you are likely to notice negative changes in your employees' work habits and behaviors. A caring co-worker may also bring an issue to your attention. Ideally, higher management or those you serve are not the ones who first bring an issue to your attention, but this is nevertheless cause for you to take action.

Act Early

Early intervention is most effective. A positive, early response heads off many serious problems and can eliminate the basis for the complaint or grievance. Many times, you can initiate a talk with the employee. Showing interest and caring for the employee helps.

Assess the Merit of the Complaint

Determine if the complaint is legitimate. The critical element in this effort is not to assume complaints are all made by whiners. Judge each complaint on its own merits.

Chronic whiners can be a problem. Consider the source as you listen and gather information. Recognize that chronic whiners enjoy causing problems. Remain objective and deal with the complaint appropriately. Making an ally of this person might be a supervisory goal.

Listen Well

Communication involves a sender, a receiver, and a message. Recognize that part of your job is receiving messages. Take the time to listen and to listen effectively. Active listening involves the use of empathy, listening, paralanguage, and body language.

To listen actively, you must pay full attention. If you do this correctly, your employee will understand that he or she has been listened to and heard. That is the essence of communication.

Listening can be difficult. Human nature prompts us to want to hear about ourselves rather than about others. Yet a supervisor needs to hear about others to be effective. Because we all listen several times faster than we speak, you may find it difficult not to interrupt or give feedback right away. It has been said that we only hear half of what is said, we listen to only half of that, and we remember only half of that. No wonder communication can be a problem.

Pay attention to paralanguage—how things are said. What is the rate of speech? What tones, inflections, and emotion are being put into what is being said? Many times how the message is delivered tells more than the actual words.

Use supportive body language. Your body language is part of your active listening. Lean in, make eye contact, use supportive gestures—these reassure the speaker that he or she is being heard. See chapter 7, on communication skills, for more on active listening.

The Resolution Process

Come to this meeting with good listening skills and a comprehensive knowledge of policy and the employee's background. If specifics of the complaint have already been made known, review this information. Your ability to resolve employee complaints and grievances hinges greatly on your skill and effectiveness in communication. The paragraphs that follow address aspects that you must effectively control.

Scheduling

Schedule adequate time for the meeting. This is not a 30-minute process. Allow time for the complaint to be heard and the discussion that needs to take place. Anticipate that a resolution will be forthcoming.

Setting

When you meet to discuss a complaint or grievance with an employee, be mindful of the location. Select an area that is private, comfortable, and free of distractions. The adage "criticize in private, praise in public" is apt. Note that private does not mean isolated and does not necessarily mean behind closed doors. Recognize that some people are uncomfortable in one-on-one meetings.

Review policies on how the meeting should take place. Some organizations require a third person to be present at any meeting that might generate a negative result. Such policies might have been designed for termination procedures, but could apply to this situation as well.

Your office is probably a poor choice for this type of meeting. You want to avoid making the employee feel isolated. Also, any plaques and awards you have on display can create a "shrine" effect and intimidate the employee.

Consider using a neutral conference room near the perimeter of the building. If the meeting proves emotional, the employee would not have to travel through the building to exit.

Documentation

Although you may need to document the process, do not let that interfere with the communication that needs to occur. Recording or taking notes can be non-productive. Instead, consider doing your documentation immediately after the meeting.

Recording especially raises major concerns and in some states is illegal without both parties' consent. Recording certainly inhibits people from expressing their feelings.

Some supervisors feel the need to take notes to accurately document what took place. If you wish to do this, obtain the employee's permission and understand that your note taking could inhibit conversation.

Tone and Attitude

Consider yourself on a fact-finding mission. You want to determine what the problem is and what the solutions are, and you want to implement a solution that is agreeable to all concerned. You want to be seen as being fair, impartial, non-judgmental, and sincerely interested in a solution. This is not much different than how you behave in any other investigation. Like other investigations, this process has a beginning, middle, and end.

Closing

If you cannot render a decision or come to a conclusion during the meeting, give the employee a reasonable expectation of when a decision will be forthcoming or what steps need to occur.

Conclusion

Resolving complaints and grievances is a critical part of employee relations. As a supervisor, you have to balance employees' needs, wants, and desires against supporting management policy and doing what is best for the organization.

First, be proactive: pay attention and be aware of what is going on in the workplace. This is how you can prevent complaints from developing. When dealing with a complaint or grievance, rely on comprehensive written policy and procedures. A successful resolution would be for the employee to return to work as a capable and productive worker. How you handle this process can determine if the outcome is positive.

Bibliography

Bintliff, R. L. 1992. *Corporate and Industrial Security*. Englewood Cliffs, NJ: Prentice Hall.

Colling, R. L. 2001. *Hospital and Healthcare Security*, 4th ed. Boston: Butterworth-Heineman.

Ouellette, R. 1993. *Management of Aggressive Behavior*. Powers Lake, Wisc: Performance Dimensions.

Wanat, J., E. Guy and J. Merrigan. 1981. *Supervisory Techniques for the Security Professional*. Boston: Butterworth.

Study and Review Questions

1. Which of the following describes a complaint?

    A. Statement of unhappiness

    B. Complaint about a process

    C. Statement about a process

    D. Complaint of unhappiness

2. Which of the following is not a stress factor?

    A. Shift work

    B. Odd or split days off

    C. Co-worker issues

    D. Desire to help people

3. How often should the employee handbook be updated?

    A. Every three years

    B. Every year

    C. Every two years

    D. Every five years

4. Which of the following is not a result of dissatisfaction?

    A. Attitude changes

    B. Tardiness

    C. Fair treatment

    D. Personality changes

5. Which of the following is not part of the resolution process?

    A. Good listening skills

    B. Comprehensive knowledge of policy

    C. Comprehensive knowledge of employee's background

    D. Time-specific discussion

Chapter 7

Communication Skills in Supervision

Dennis Parr, CHPA, CPP

OBJECTIVES

After studying this chapter, the student should understand the following:

- Active listening skills
- Barriers to effective listening
- Core conditions of effective communications
- Meeting management
- Effective writing skills
- Ten critical business-writing problems
- Effective e-mail writing

Adults with successful careers, happy personal lives, and lasting friendships have something in common: they know how to communicate effectively. The ability to interact properly with others is one of the most powerful tools to use for ensuring professional and personal success. Security directors, program managers, supervisors, and all officers must possess good communication skills.

As a supervisor, your day is full of events requiring communication—interviewing suspects, witnesses, and new security employees; resolving complaints; discussing issues with your manager. In each interaction, the communication (listening, speaking, and writing) can make or break your day. One of the surest ways to alienate yourself from others is to communicate poorly. The way a message is communicated can be more important than the message itself. Effective communication skills are simple, and you can learn them by consciously using and practicing them. Developing these skills helps you become an effective leader.

Listening

Good listening is an unnatural act. If it were not, we would see more of it around. Conflict and emotion exist in all human interactions and affect each person differently.

Developing Emotional Intelligence

Your emotional intelligence is your ability to control your behaviors and emotions in relationships with others. The ability to manage emotion and conflict often results from habits and styles developed early in life. Well-honed emotional intelligence is critical to success in any area of life. In interpersonal relationships, the person with the most flexibility in behavior always has the upper hand. Conversely, limiting your behavior allows others to get the competitive edge. Behavior and emotion are interrelated and cannot exist without each other. Timing is also of utmost importance.

Emotions impact reasoning, and lingering negative emotions always derail the best efforts. Becoming more aware of your emotions and those of others helps you control your emotions and thus achieve emotional intelligence. This understanding leads to control and increased ability to adapt and respond to all situations.

Smart Sending and Receiving

Understanding is bi-directional:

- *As the sender*, use all means possible to make certain your message is understood
- *As the receiver*, do everything possible to receive and understand the intended message

In other words, to be an effective communicator, you must learn to listen as well as to speak and to write.

Promoting Understanding. Concerning anything said or heard, you must continually watch for any possible points of misunderstanding and clarify any ambiguity. Asking for confirmation includes rephrasing what the speaker said. Below are some reasons mis-understandings can occur. Be on the lookout for these.

- ***Lacking Context:*** Words often have different meanings, based upon the context used and upon culture. For example, a "funny" incident can be either amusing or troubling. When speaking with others, give background for context. When listening to others, ask questions to establish context in your own mind.
- ***Error in Word Choice:*** Mistakes are sometimes made in the choice of words used. The solution is to recognize ambiguities and resolve inconsistencies.
- ***Mis-heard:*** Sometimes, people simply incorrectly hear what is being said. Omission of a single word can change the entire meaning of a statement.

Planning to be Effective. As with all effective communication, planning can eliminate many communication problems. Decide on the purpose of a conversation and plan how to achieve that purpose. This helps you remove many communication challenges.

Conflicts are sometimes painful because they often remain unresolved. When the parties seek to resolve the conflict—and handle it correctly—seeing the opposite side can be an eye-opener, sometimes even a life-changing opportunity.

Using Active Listening Skills

The position of your head and your facial expressions, in addition to other forms of body language, communicate emotions such as interest, disagreement, surprise, or humor. Active listening involves physically using your head and eyes to communicate listening. The sidebar lists active listening skills you should be using. These "attending" skills let the speaker know that you are interested in what is being said.

Active Listening Skills
- ***Engaged Body Language:*** When people desire to communicate effectively, they turn physically toward each other, lean slightly forward, and maintain eye contact. Use this attentive body language to convey interest and remove distracting barriers.
- ***Reassuring Eye Contact:*** Attentive listeners maintain varied eye contact. Do not stare, but maintain eye contact approximately 80 percent of the time.
- ***Verbal Interaction:*** Ask questions to encourage the speaker to continue speaking and to give more details. There are two ways of phrasing questions: (1) open-ended questions and (2) closed questions. An open-ended question forces the person answering to relate more information. Asking "How have you handled this problem in the past?" (open-ended question) gives you more information than asking, "Have you encountered this problem before?" (closed question).
- ***Active Listening:*** Once the person is talking, the other person's job is to listen. Listening is the most important skill a good communicator can master. It is the core of good communications.

Inattentive Listening Behaviors
- Starting to argue
- Looking away or looking upward
- Showing an expression of disagreement
- Shaking the head
- Arching the eyebrows
- Folding the arms
- Leaning back
- Looking ready to speak

Chapter 7: Communication Skills in Supervision

Below is an example of effective listening:

You: Tell me how the new revised form we began using last Monday is working for you.
The Other: Well, the form seems to be useful, but at times it is confusing.
You: It's useful but also confusing?
The Other: Yes, it is hard to know what some of the questions are really asking for.
You: Some of the questions are vague or confusing?
The Other: Yes, especially questions 4 and 18.
You: Those questions seem to be particularly confusing?
The Other: Yes, and I think it is because they do not refer to anything that has been said previously.

You can see that the listener has simply listened to what the speaker has said and responded by reflecting back, sometimes paraphrasing, almost exactly what the other person has said. Contrast that effective style of listening with an example of poor listening:

You: How is the new revised form we began using last week going?
The Other: Well, it seems to be going okay, but some of it is kind of confusing.
You: Well, I guess you just have to use it for a while longer, and it will probably start to iron out.
The Other: Some of the questions are really hard to understand.
You: Maybe if you went back and read them again very carefully, they would start to make sense to you.
The Other: Some of the questions are okay, but a few are difficult to understand.
You: We really spent a lot of time writing those questions, and I think they are pretty clear.

The second conversation indicates that the listener is really not listening to what the speaker is saying. Rather, the "listener" is preparing an argument—to defend the work already done. In the first instance (good listening), the speaker probably came away feeling heard and understood by the other person. In effect, the speaker was validated. In the second example (demonstrating poor listening skills), the speaker probably went away feeling frustrated and somewhat angry. The speaker tried to say something, but was undercut and distracted by the responses of the listener.

If You Are Not Being Listened to, Stop and Listen

Talking to someone who is not listening is a waste of time for both parties. A way to help the listener become more receptive to what is being said is to skillfully listen to that person first. Once the individual feels heard, he or she is more likely to listen to what you are saying.

Learn to recognize inattentive listening behaviors. See the sidebar earlier in this chapter for some common ones. If you are talking and see that the other person is no longer listening, quickly stop talking and switch to listening mode. Say something like, "You do not seem to agree with what I am saying..." and then listen for the response.

Using Silence

As an information-gathering strategy, silence can be quite effective, especially in investigations and interrogations. The technique is used less frequently than it should be.

Many people are nervous with silence; they feel they must fill the void. Thus, when you are seeking information, try silence. Ask your question and wait for the person to answer. Nod, smile, and keep silent while you wait. The person will likely give more details simply to fill the ensuing silence.

Barriers to Effective Listening

Learn to recognize obstacles to effective listening. Are you creating any of the barriers listed on the next page in the sidebar? Are important communications from you hampered by any of these obstacles?

Barriers to Effective Listening

- *Dovetailing:* When someone is talking and the listener agrees with the speaker by saying, "I really agree with what you have to say because of the experience I just had...", this agreement can derail what the first person was saying.

- *Arguing:* If the listener begins to argue (disagree) with the speaker, this can sidetrack or discourage the speaker.

- *Over-reacting:* An emotional over-reaction can prevent effective listening. Gasping and crying out in dismay are examples of over-reacting behaviors that can be observed in conversations between managers and employees.

- *Distracting Behavior:* People sometimes engage in distracting behaviors such as tapping their fingers, shuffling through papers, rocking in their chairs, or glancing frequently at a clock. Such distractions can stop the effective flow of communication.

- *Questioning:* Interrupting with questions can sometimes pose a barrier to effective listening. If someone starts to talk about hospital policy and is suddenly asked who wrote the policy, the speaker will have to answer the question posed, rather than talk about an interesting event that happened on the campus. A listener should only ask questions about information that is truly needed and only ask the question when it does not sidetrack the speaker.

Core Conditions of Effective Communication

These four variables seem to be common in effective communication:

- Accurate empathy
- Positive regard
- Genuineness
- Specificity

Accurate Empathy

Accurate empathy is the ability to go beyond the spoken message and identify with and understand another's situation, feelings, and motives. What a speaker says about his or her feelings is not always accurate.

For example, if a speaker says, "I do not care," but at the same time slams a palm sharply on the tabletop and frowns, the message is probably not, "I do not care." The speaker probably cares greatly and may be angry or upset.

You can offer what seems to be a more accurate reflection of the message by saying, "You seem angry about this." This effective response is neither a simple reflection of the words used nor a question. You are stating what you perceive to be the actual message of the speaker. You are accurately reflecting the message, without embellishment.

Positive Regard

Whether they agree or disagree, two communicators must have a basic level of unconditional positive regard for one another. If they do not, communication is, by definition, strained. All this really means is that the two parties must have "good will" toward each other. Good will has to be present for effective communication to occur.

Genuineness

To be genuine is to be sincere, not fake, and to be honest and open. Most people can easily sense when the other party is not being genuine. The person might verbally agree or nod and appear to be listening, but the total message conveyed, verbally and non-verbally, clearly is not genuine.

A good communicator's response to the other person is genuine. Do not confuse tactlessness and brutal honesty with being genuine. Also, avoid "game playing." Focus on expressing your true and accurate response in a genuine way.

Specificity
An effective communicator tries to be specific and use voice references (tone, speed, inflection) that make sense when speaking. Just as the listener tries to follow along with what the other person is saying, the speaker tries to follow along exactly with what the conversation is about. When the listener responds to what is said, the reply needs to be as specific as possible.

For example, "oh, really" is not as specific as, "what you are talking about is your disagreement with what was said on the night of March 24." The first statement is not specific, and the second is very specific. This specificity clarifies the details needed.

At the end of a conversation, confirm clear understanding of the outcome. For example, if a decision was made, repeat what should happen and the timeline. If questions have been asked, summarize what has been learned.

Meeting Management

As with every other managed activity, meetings should be planned in advance, monitored for effectiveness as they take place, and reviewed afterward for improvement. A meeting is the ultimate form of managed conversation.

Chairing
Chairing a meeting signifies organizing the information and meeting structure to facilitate effective communication of the participants. Meetings should only be held when needed, and only those who need to attend and have something to contribute should be invited. An ending time for the meeting should be specified so everyone is aware and can plan their time accordingly.

The Agenda
An agenda sent out in advance of the meeting informs participants of the subject and organizes discussion at the meeting. Circulating a draft agenda and asking for additional topics that need to be covered both informs participants in advance and solicits ideas. Before the meeting starts, a revised agenda should be sent with enough time for people to prepare their contributions.

Conduct
Establishing a code of conduct or rules of order is essential for effective meetings. Some companies post these in meeting rooms so all participants are reminded to follow them. The following expectations are usually part of the rules of order:

- Respect the opinions of others
- Adhere to time limits
- Arrive on time

The confidence with which individuals participate often determines the success of a meeting. All ideas should be welcomed, and no one should ever be laughed at or disregarded. Avoid and discourage direct criticism of any person. Be sure to identify and follow up on all action items to increase effectiveness.

Effective Writing

The mechanics of written communications (e.g., reports, investigations, e-mails) are often ignored. The difference between a well-written document and a poorly written one can dramatically affect an organization and cost a great deal in time and money. When writing is ineffective, readers may miss the good ideas or discount them. Anyone can learn and follow the basic steps of effective writing.

The need to be precise increases as the technical content of the material grows. The tremendous growth of information technology has not reduced the need for effective written communication. This explosion has actually added more issues for concern for writers since the means for communication have increased and become more complex.

Writing is not simply the process of putting words on paper or on a computer screen. Writing is situational and persuasive. Writing requires understanding the audience, the correct timing, and the readers' culture. Effective writing, therefore, involves analysis, organization, and planning.

Writing should serve a purpose; otherwise, the material need not be written. When planning to write, seek to answer pertinent questions, such as who, what, where, when, why, and how.

Ten Critical Business-writing Problems
Ten serious problems common in business writing are listed in the sidebar. Analyze your written communications for these so you do not lessen the impact of your work.

Ten Critical Problems in Business Writing
1. Inadequate organization
2. Incorrect spelling and capitalization
3. Improper punctuation and grammar
4. Misused words
5. Redundancy
6. Unnecessary words
7. Lengthy paragraphs
8. Lengthy sentences
9. Passive language
10. Inappropriate tone

Source: Blake, G. 3 Apr 1995. It is recommended that you write clearly. *Wall Street Journal*, pA14(W) pA16(E), col 4.

Audience Needs
Different readers have different needs, and as a writer, you must relate the material to those specific needs. A reader must quickly perceive the benefits of reading the document; therefore, you must keep in mind how the reader will interpret and process the information.

Target Audience. Before you begin writing, consider the following about the target audience:
- Needs
- Attitudes
- Backgrounds
- Level of understanding

Tailor the message to fit those characteristics. Doing so produces more effective communication.

Organization
Maximize the effectiveness of your communication by attending to the following details regarding its organization.

- **Introduction:** A solid introduction is essential. Spend more time preparing this than any other part of the document. Since some readers only read the first paragraph, you must not only convey a great deal of information, but effectively convince the reader to continue reading.
- **Main Points:** Know the main points and, very early in the document, make them clear.
- **Supports:** Follow each key point with the rationale or supporting details.
- **Chunking:** Group complex or technical material into manageable and logical sections. Doing so provides a "map" for the reader to follow in understanding what is being written. Failure to present complex information clearly may confuse and frustrate readers.
- **Transitions:** Use transition sentences to enable the reader to understand the shift from one topic to another.

Format and Style
Once you have the material organized, shift your focus to making a straightforward presentation. Consider the document's format and your writing style. In terms of writing style, you want to "keep it short and simple," which you can remember with the acronym KISS. Provide numerous clues, through the document's format, so readers know what they should do as they read this communication.

- **Headings:** Use headings and subheadings as "road markers" to aid clarity.
- **Paragraphing:** Make each paragraph a group of closely related sentences "bundled" for manageability. All sentences within paragraphs should branch out from and support a main idea.

- **Topic Sentences:** Use the first or second sentence of the paragraph to indicate its main topic. The topic sentence is a kind of label for the paragraph and should indicate the contents for the remainder of the paragraph.
- **Readability:** Use bullets, tables, charts, and graphics, as appropriate, to improve the appearance and readability of the writing.
- **Length**: Most memos should consist of no more than one paragraph, and a letter should be no longer than three paragraphs. All proposals and reports should have a summary at the very beginning that is no longer than two pages.

Brevity. To finalize the writing, scan it again to ensure appropriate conciseness. Look for unnecessary words and delete these. This last step usually involves eliminating some adverbs and adjectives, flowery and poetic words, and everything else that is unnecessary or wordy. Strip the message down to the "bare bones" so anyone can read it clearly and enjoy the simple message being sent. Below is an example of a memo that is wordy and pretentious.

To: All Managers of the Management Team
From: The Security Director
Regarding: Mandatory Management Meeting

This message is to inform you that there will be a mandatory meeting for all members of the management team to discuss the implications of having an outside consulting firm come into our organization to consult with us on the feasibility of utilizing a marketing strategy and to plan expansion of our high-potential stock items. All managers of the management team are required to attend this meeting at 9:00 a.m. Tuesday, December 12 in Conference Room B-1.

You can see that this memo is not only wordy and pretentious, but also uses many large words where simple ones would suffice. See if you can edit this into simpler text.

Here is how the message could be improved by eliminating the excess verbiage:

To: All Managers
From: Security Director
Regarding: Meeting with Marketing Consulting Firm

Please attend a meeting on Tuesday, December 12, at 9 am in Conference Room B-1 to discuss our planned sales expansion with a marketing consulting firm.

Notice the big difference in these two messages. Of course, you have to consider how short you want your message to be. If you feel you have to convince your audience to do something and need to load up the beginning with a persuasive pitch, then do so. Make your pitch simple and straightforward. Since the memo in the example is from a director, starting with a simple first-person invitation might get the reader's attention. If the director felt a need to convince managers of the importance of this meeting, a sentence could be added to stress this. However, much of that can be conducted via face-to-face contact, rather than through memos.

Effective E-mails

E-mail costs less and is faster than a letter, less interruption than a telephone call, and less bother than a fax. Using e-mail makes differences in location and time zone less of an obstacle. Because of these advantages, e-mail use has exploded. Its speed and broadcasting ability make electronic communication fundamentally different from paper-based communication. Since its turnaround time can be very fast, e-mail tends to be more conversational than traditional paper-based communication.

In a paper document, all writing must be clear and unambiguous, since the intended audience may not have a chance to ask for clarification. E-mail documents allow the recipient to ask questions immediately in a reply e-mail. E-mail, therefore, (just like conversational speech) tends to be less precise than paper communications.

E-mail does not convey emotions as well as face-to-face conversations or even telephone conversations. E-mail communication does not contain vocal inflections or gestures; thus, the receiver may have difficulty ascertaining if the writer is serious or joking. Sarcasm is particularly dangerous in e-mail communications.

Subject Line

In e-mails, the writer must be careful to put the message in context. The subject line is one way to set this up. A subject line pertaining clearly to the body of the e-mail assists readers in placing the message in the proper context. Make the subject line short, but indicative of the message's content. For time-critical messages, begin the subject line with the word "URGENT," especially if the reader receives many e-mails.

Formatting

Avoid elaborate formatting. Some e-mail reading software only understands plain text. Text in italics, bold, and color may look unusual or may show up as characters (< or >) in the text. Web documents are particularly difficult to read using older e-mail software programs. To minimize problems, keep the receiver's computer capabilities in mind (whenever possible) when sending Web pages as text or as documents formatted in HTML (hypertext markup language).

Links

Some e-mail reading software recognizes URLs (Uniform Resource Locators, or Web addresses) in the text and makes them "live" (able to take the reader directly to that Web site by clicking on them with the mouse). Other software may not recognize links and may only allow the reader to "cut and paste" the link into the Web address area.

Attachments

Most mailers support file attachments (documents sent with the e-mail). Be aware that recipients will be unable to open the attachment or unable to view it in the correct format if they do not have the software with which it was created. Even if the recipient can receive and view the attachment, problems can occur if the file attachment is too large. Large attachments could cause the recipient's computer to be low on disk space or take a tiresome amount of time to open if the recipient has only a dial-up connection.

If you are unaware of what e-mail reader recipients use, employ these tips:

- Avoid using formatted text
- Be aware of special characters
- Enter Web pages as text
- Before URLs, type in "http://"
- Be careful when sending attachments

Length

E-mail paragraphs should be shortened to only a few sentences each, since they may be read in a document window with scrollbars. Scrollbars make it harder to visually read long paragraphs. Word wrapping within the software can also create problems.

Emotion

Emotion is difficult to communicate in e-mails. Without the tone of voice to indicate the emotion, the reader can easily mis-interpret the intent. You can use capital letters, asterisks, or exclamation points to convey emphasis. Be judicious, though: using all capital letters can indicate extreme emphasis. Some people represent facial gestures as "smiley faces" or "emoticons," but you should use these only in very informal e-mails. Examples are ☺ or ☹.

Tone

The tone and formality of an e-mail determines how many responses it receives. Chatty and informal e-mails encourage readers to respond. A more formal style discourages readers from sending a response.

Impression

Just as with any written communication, recipients make assumptions about the writer based on e-mails. Mis-spelled words, grammar mistakes, or punctuation errors may lead a recipient to infer that you are uneducated or do not pay enough attention to detail. Even though e-mail communication is more informal, proofreading is still important. Use grammar and spell checkers to avoid making negative impressions.

Etiquette

Not everyone within an organization is privileged to have an e-mail address or mailbox. Those who have them should use them, particularly in replying to e-mails sent by others. People may be accustomed to calling on the telephone or going to see someone in person, as they did before getting an e-mail address. Unless there is a reason for not communicating via e-mail, that is the preferred method in many instances.

When sending time-critical e-mails, be proactive to ensure you get the response you need. Contact the party in another way (e.g., phone) to point out the significance of the e-mail.

Group Lists

Group lists are easy to establish for sending e-mails to a group of people. Group notifications are an excellent means of communicating with large numbers of people at once; however, take care to use the "reply to all" feature sparingly. Always remember that when you reply to all instead of to just one party, everyone on the list has to take time to read the response.

Privacy and Security

Using e-mail requires you, and your staff and those with whom you communicate, to be aware of the privacy and security issues this technology raises.

- Once given an e-mail address, protect that e-mail address and only share it with those who have reasons to communicate via e-mail.

- Protect your e-mail inbox at all times. When stepping away from your computer, either lock the computer screen or exit the e-mail program.

- Be mindful that personal information you divulge in the signature line is provided to all recipients; exercise caution in sharing this information or forwarding the personal information of others.

Conclusion

The Bible tells of the tower of Babel, which collapsed because people were no longer able to communicate. Speech became so varied that people could no longer understand one another. Could today's communications forms disable you? Without specific effort, your conversation and writing become ineffective. As a supervisor, you must treat a conversation or written document like any other managed activity:

- Establish a purpose
- Plan ahead
- Verify that the purpose has been achieved

Bibliography

Alred, G. J., C. T. Brusaw and W. E. Olie. 2006. *The Business Writer's Handbook*, 8th ed. New York: St. Martin's Press.

Colling, R. L. 2001. *Hospital and Healthcare Security*, 4th ed. Boston: Butterworth-Heinemann.

Covey, S. R. 1989. *The Seven Habits of Highly Effective People*. New York: Simon and Schuster.

Study and Review Questions

1. What type of act is listening?

- *A.* Unnatural
- *B.* Natural
- *C.* Intuitive
- *D.* Emotional

2. What type of questions should you use to gather information?

- *A.* Closed
- *B.* Open-ended
- *C.* Short and to the point
- *D.* Forceful

3. Which of the following is not a core condition of effective communications?

- *A.* Accurate empathy
- *B.* Positive regard
- *C.* Free of distraction
- *D.* Genuineness

4. The first part of organizing writing is what?

- *A.* Complex material
- *B.* Formatting
- *C.* Style
- *D.* Solid introduction

5. Which of the following is not an advantage of e-mail?

- *A.* Costs less
- *B.* Faster than a letter
- *C.* More of an interruption than a phone call
- *D.* Less of a bother than a fax

Chapter 8

Self-improvement

Bonnie S. Michelman, CPP, CHPA

OBJECTIVES

After studying this chapter, the student should understand the following:

- The importance of continual self-improvement
- How to make and use a personal inventory of habits, attitudes, and traits
- How to set broad personal goals and objectives to attain those goals
- How to establish action plans to reach personal goals
- Improvements to maximize the work effort of subordinates
- Proven strategies for gaining recognition and achievement on the job

Self-improvement is essential to your success. The process by which you improve your performance and skills is neither dull nor standardized. This ongoing initiative always requires new effort, and you create the roadmap—a custom-designed self-improvement plan that reflects your abilities and personality. As you strive to improve your performance and skills as a supervisor, remember that your primary job as a supervisor is maximizing the effort of each employee you supervise—rather than doing the tasks assigned to your employees. Consider the following as you develop your personal improvement program: your physical and mental condition, your morals, your personal relationships, and your current supervisory skills and duties.

Self-awareness

Knowing and being aware of your strong and weak points helps you establish realistic goals and objectives and allows you to succeed in your efforts. The first step—the one you need to make before you will see any improvements—is to properly identify your current skills and abilities through a self-assessment. After completing this assessment, you determine which skills you want to improve. Finally, you implement a plan to make the desired improvements.

This chapter provides a few sample assessment tools, but you are strongly urged to use additional resources. One is Stephen Covey's *Seven Habits of Highly Effective People*.

Self-evaluation

- Honestly assess yourself—Recognize your talents
- Have your performance assessed—Use your supervisor's insights
- Mentor and be mentored—Share your experience and expertise, and learn in the process

Self-improvement Inventory for Supervisors

Answer these questions honestly to obtain a reliable self-assessment.

Please make a copy of this inventory for personal use. Retain the checklist in the book as a master.

Performance Characteristic	Current Status (circle one)	Areas to Improve (✓)	Priorities (highest, medium, lowest)	Anticipated Date to Reach Related Goal	Comments
Do I inspire desired actions from my subordinates?	Yes No Sometimes				
Do I share not only the criticism but, more importantly, the praise my subordinates deserve?	Yes No Sometimes				
Do I set a good example with my work ethics, initiative, optimism and enthusiasm?	Yes No Sometimes				
Am I attentive to details?	Yes No Sometimes				
Do I have and display confidence in myself?	Yes No Sometimes				
Do I recognize and acknowledge accomplishments of others (subordinates)?	Yes No Sometimes				
Do I keep abreast of developments in my field?	Yes No Sometimes				
Do I have and display a genuine interest in people?	Yes No Sometimes				
Do I really listen to what others have to say and give deserved consideration to their ideas?	Yes No Sometimes				
Am I fair in my dealings with others?	Yes No Sometimes				
Do I keep myself mentally and physically fit?	Yes No Sometimes				
Do I assume responsibility for my actions?	Yes No Sometimes				
Do I inspire team action?	Yes No Sometimes				
Do I give clear and complete instructions?	Yes No Sometimes				
Do I set realistic goals for myself and for others?	Yes No Sometimes				
Do I display a calm demeanor under adverse conditions?	Yes No Sometimes				
Am I tolerant of other people's morals, feelings, and customs?	Yes No Sometimes				
Do I exert positive leadership?	Yes No Sometimes				
Am I successful at achieving my goals?	Yes No Sometimes				
Do I display a non-prejudiced attitude toward individuals and groups?	Yes No Sometimes				

Self-improvement Inventory for Supervisors

Copy the self-improvement inventory in this book. Complete the checklist, and review your answers. As you might expect, the desired answer to each question is "yes." Consider any question to which you cannot truthfully answer "yes" an area you should improve.

After identifying your strong and weak points, you can (1) take full advantage of your positive skills and (2) begin to change your less desirable traits. You will probably be more successful if you focus on one habit or trait at a time until you meet that goal. Make periodic progress checks and adjustments to your plan as you grow and your needs change.

Setting and Achieving Goals

Broad Goals

Goals are a rough roadmap of where you want to be. The goals you set should be general in nature (e.g., to listen to others and consider their opinions). Each goal should have an approximate completion date (e.g., 6 months, 1 year).

Specific Objectives

To reach your goals, you need to set objectives. The objectives detail the specific actions you will take to reach the goal. Think of the objectives as steps along your path to success. Assign a specific, expected completion date to each objective you define. This helps keep you motivated and on track.

Your Written Plan

When written clearly and specifically, defined objectives and timelines keep you focused on your desired results. As you select your goals and objectives and put them on paper, note (1) who you need to help you take these steps and (2) the resources (e.g., books, reports, data) you require. Define the start date and anticipated completion date of each objective, as one objective often depends on the completion of another.

The table shown is one method of documenting both your plan and your progress. Sample entries are provided only as examples.

Goal What I Want to Do	Objectives Steps to Accomplish Goal	Resources Needed	Timeline (date started: date to be completed)
Improve skills in human relations: managing conflicts	Pick a college course Discuss with my supervisor Register for the course	Course catalogs Adjust work schedule Financial assistance	Nov 1: Spring semester
Increase knowledge of effective supervision	1 Buy and read Covey's book 2 Establish my goals and objectives 3 Meet with security director to review my performance evaluation 4 Attend IAHSS supervisor training	1 Resource book 2 Time to read resource book and complete charts 3 Copy of all prior evaluations 4 Register for and attend next supervisor program	Sep 4: Oct 4 Oct 11: Oct 18 Oct 20: Oct 21 Oct 28: Nov 14
Spend more time interacting with my family	Plan family vacation Schedule home time More books, less TV	Cash in savings bonds Plan 1 family meal/day Go to book store	Sep 6: Sep 20 Sep 4 Sep 4: Sep 6

Reaching Your Goals

The following general guidelines may be helpful for your program of personal development as a security supervisor:

- Analyze your current position. Learn from your mistakes and your successes.

- Review and learn duties and responsibilities of others to improve your skills.

- Seek additional responsibility. If comfortable handling present duties and you feel you can handle more tasks or responsibility, request them.

- Set realistic goals that are beneficial to you *and* possible for you to accomplish.

- Seek educational benefits on or off the job. Adding educational credentials to your list of personal assets (be they academic, supervisory, or other job-specific courses) contributes to your self-development. The better educated and trained you are, the more valuable you are to your organization.

- Continually review and modify your plan. As your situation or your opportunities change, your plan will need periodic revision (at least yearly).

Goal setting should be an ongoing process. Setting personal, employment, and social goals is the impetus to self-improvement. Reaching a goal—whether it is improving a work habit, completing a course of study, or getting to know and understand others—creates great feelings of accomplishment.

Working with Others

You no doubt have found that some of the people you must deal with on a daily basis can be "difficult." In working with others, always remember we each seek to accomplish tasks and goals in the ways in which we are most familiar. Since most people are not mirror images of each other (which is probably a good thing), you have to be able to "deal with" others. As a supervisor, you need this ability for two reasons: to elicit maximum performance from those you supervise and to benefit from those who supervise you. You need to know which approach will obtain the best results. For example, should you be a strict disciplinarian or approach the person as a fellow team member?

Brandon Toropov offers some guidance in his book *The Complete Idiot's Guide to Getting Along with Difficult People*. Toropov suggests that we are likely to describe any person who does not do things "the way we want them to" as a difficult person, while in fact we may be the difficult one. He also suggests that once you accept that the other person is different and begin to acknowledge the good things that person does, you establish some common ground and diminish the difficulty.

All people are motivated by success (what works for them). If their methods are different from ours (even if the desired results are obtained), we are likely to describe them as difficult.

For example, you assign a subordinate to tally a specific set of statistics, but that person refuses to use an adding machine even though you said it was required to minimize possible mistakes. You might describe that person as difficult even though that person is a math whiz and can add faster and more accurately without the adding machine. To remove the feeling that someone is being difficult, find a suitable common ground on which you can both function. For example, suggest spot checks with an adding machine; then, if no errors are noted, no adding machine will be required.

Remember, as a supervisor you are not going to—nor will you have to—like all the personalities in your work relationships. You are, however, expected to learn enough about personalities to adapt your supervisory technique for each person under your charge. Become familiar with the keys to success in forming successful teams, remind yourself of ways to overcome resistance, and learn to work despite conflict. Pointers on each of these topics are given on the next page.

Forming Successful Teams

The following are keys to success in working on teams:

- Clear mission and vision—Why does your organization and team exist?
- Written goals
- Clear purpose—Daily, weekly, monthly, quarterly
- High level of participation
- Ability to resolve conflict
- Ability to reach consensus
- Strong and frequent communication—Top down, bottom up
- Shared responsibility
- Shared leadership
- Appreciation of diversity

Overcoming Resistance to Change

Here are five smart tactics for overcoming resistance to change:

- Let people know as far in advance as possible
- Ask team members for input
- Confront anxiety or negativity privately with team members
- Address "what's in it for me?"—Personally, team, department, organization
- Redefine job role and responsibility

Overcoming Discomfort with Conflict

If you are uncomfortable with conflict, periodically remind yourself of the following:

- Conflict is a healthy signal that something needs attention.
- You cannot consider alternatives that do not exist. When handled properly, reasonable conflict can function as an "idea generator."
- Look at conflicting viewpoints as intellectual or procedural "sparring partners."
- Let the other party save face unless you want to start a "revenge account" that earns compound interest.
- Remember, the quality of the solution and acceptance by you and your staff are the goals. If your strategy does not lead toward that kind of solution, re-examine your strategy and motives immediately.

Developing a Leader's Perspective

As you strive to improve your ability to work with and lead others more effectively, Toropov's "least you need to know" list may be some help:

- All of us have preferences for either team or independent work
- Some of us work for timelines, some for perfection
- Subordinates respond best in situations where they feel their preferences are being supported
- Public criticism, even with no names, is de-motivating
- You really can develop a skill, or bring it into existence, through the use of praise
- Getting subordinates involved in planning gives them a feeling of ownership and participation
- Chronic complainers may make great quality control people
- Setting and maintaining appropriate standards for workplace speech is essential
- Some employees live to make everyone else's life miserable—the best thing you can do is observe and follow appropriate legal and organizational safeguards as appropriate for terminating their employment

Managing change has become a critical responsibility of leaders in today's organizations. Your role as a leader is to provide a stabilizing influence as changes occur.

Outcomes of Self-improvement

The true gain you realize from self-improvement is in your personal worth; however, specific job-related improvements may also occur. For example:

- Enhanced job performance
- Increased employee morale
- Increased employee efficiency
- Increased professionalism
- Better understanding of others
- Positive, objective attitudes for you and others
- Improved setting and achieving of goals
- Promotion

Strategies That Promote Job Advancement

The eight strategies listed in the sidebar are key in career advancement. The results of your efforts will become visible to all your fellow employees and your supervisors. When advancement opportunity knocks, you will be there—ready, willing, and able to accept the new duties. Opportunities may exist in your own department, in other areas of the organization, or even in another facility. As you develop and display the self-confidence needed to climb the next rung on the success ladder, you will be viewed as someone who can.

Eight "P"s to Job Advancement

Positive thinking—about your potential
- Project yourself—visualize a success scenario
- Program yourself to realize your vision

Progressive ideas—for work improvement
- Present innovative ideas to your manager
- Publicize yourself; let others know your ideas
- Persuade supervisors to accept your suggestions; be assertive
- Put your ideas into action

Problem-solving ability
- Proactively solve problems—resolve problems rather than complain about them
- Promote an attitude of seeking solutions versus placing blame

Priorities for your time and your tasks
- Place first things first; prioritize tasks daily
- Practice good time management

People skills
- Plan periodic positive interactions with superiors; learn how to manage your manager
- Practice effective human relations with subordinates
- Put open, two-way communications into practice

Participative management
- Permit people to take self-generating action, share, and collaborate
- Prepare people to move ahead—so you can move ahead

Proactive performance
- Push ahead with what needs doing; accept extra responsibility
- Produce—promotions go to the productive

Planning—for advancement
- Put your self-improvement goals into effect

Professional Growth and Development

Professional growth and development go hand in hand with self-improvement. These are ongoing processes. When and if they end, you go backward.

Anticipating Change

Working in an organization, you must be on the lookout for change. Anticipate that the people around you and the organization itself are constantly evolving. Frequently reconsider what you may need to do differently in response to the current environment. Recognize that time does not stand still: all aspects of your organization, the job, and what is expected of you continually change.

Personnel Changes. Fellow employees and supervisors come and go. When this happens, the efforts required for establishing and maintaining effective relationships and networks become even more important. If your relationships stagnate, cooperation suffers and the working environment becomes stressful and tense. Every new person coming on the job requires that you establish a new and different effective working relationship.

Changes in the Work Environment. Organizational and regulatory rules, instructions, and policies as well as laws are in constant flux. You have the responsibility to keep up on new developments to more effectively complete your job. Facilities change as new buildings are built or areas are renovated. These necessitate changes in patrols, post, and all related assignments. You must be aware of these changes since the protection of property remains a key responsibility.

Changes Outside of Work. Change also occurs in our personal lives. The attitudes and skills discussed in this chapter can help you deal with changes in your personal life as well.

Conclusion

Your job consumes a large portion of your life. Thus, you should attempt to make your work as enjoyable and profitable as possible. Your enjoyment of this work is directly related to your abilities to work with and supervise others. Your ability to adapt to and prepare for the changes that will continually occur—not only at work, but also in your personal life—becomes extremely important.

Self-improvement is a never-ending process that requires your constant attention. Your efforts will be most effective when you follow a set plan with established goals and objectives. Effective self-improvement results in the development of improved personal and professional relationships and provides you with maximum economic and psychological rewards.

Bibliography

Colling, R. L. 2001. *Hospital and Healthcare Security,* 4th ed. Boston: Butterworth-Heinemann.

Covey, S. R. 1994. *First Things First.* New York: Free Press.

Dowell, C. 2004. "Self Improvement." In *Supervisory Training Manual and Study Guide for Healthcare Security Personnel* (E. Meserve, ed.). Glendale Heights, Ill: International Association for Healthcare Security and Safety.

Toropov, B. 1997. *The Complete Idiot's Guide to Getting Along with Difficult People.* Indianapolis: Alpha Books.

Study and Review Questions

1. Which of the following is not a step of self-evaluation?

    A. Honestly assess yourself

    B. Have your performance assessed

    C. Listen to your best friend's assessment

    D. Mentor and be mentored

2. Which of the following best describes the definition of goals?

    A. Rough roadmap of where you want to be

    B. Specific roadmap of where you want to be

    C. General objectives

    D. Specific idea of where you want to be

3. What type of process is goal setting?

    A. Short-term

    B. Ongoing

    C. One-time

    D. Long-term

4. Which of the following is not an outcome of self-improvement?

    A. Enhanced job performance

    B. Increased professionalism

    C. Better understanding of others

    D. Less employee efficiency

5. What is a common thread in professional growth and development?

    A. Continual change

    B. Stagnant relationships

    C. Stagnant cooperation

    D. Minor change

Chapter 9

Civil Liability and the Supervisor

Tony W. York, MBA, MS, CHPA, CPP

OBJECTIVES

After studying this chapter, the student should understand the following:

- Basics of our legal system
- Key legal concepts
- The four elements of a tort and the two burdens of proof
- How and to whom civil liability may attach
- How supervisors should perform their work to minimize the healthcare organization's liability exposure and the supervisor's personal liability exposure
- Significant legal issues in the employment relationship
- The relationship between management decisions and legal considerations
- The importance of good documentation and the disciplinary process

---

Notice: The information in this chapter is general in nature and has been designed to serve as a guide to facilitate learning and discussion. This material is not to be construed as the direct rendering of legal or management advice. If you have a specific need or problem, seek the services of competent legal counsel or other appropriate professionals.

Please see the list of key terms at the end of this chapter for the definition of any term shown in **bold** within a paragraph.

When beginning to learn about civil liability, your first questions might be these: Where do I find the law? In what books do I look? How do I learn what I can and cannot do? Unfortunately, you will find no easy answers. The law is found in many forms and places. As background for this discussion, let's look first at what makes up the law in the United States.

The Law: An Introduction

The US Constitution
The US Constitution, as ratified by the original thirteen states, created the federal government, gave the federal government certain powers, and required that all subsequently enacted federal and state laws comply with the Constitution. Because no law may offend (or disagree with) it, the Constitution is referred to as the "supreme law of the land."

States' Rights
All power and authority not given to the federal government is reserved by the states. As a result, each state has its own Constitution. State constitutions create the state government and give the state government all powers and authority not given to the federal government.

Included among these reserved rights is the right to provide *even greater protection* (than does the US Constitution or federal law) to people within each state's jurisdiction.

Comparing the Federal and State Systems
Under our constitutional system, two bodies of law are constantly developing side by side: federal law and state law. Many similarities exist between our federal and state systems. For example, both systems have three equal branches:

- *Executive Branch:* Enforces the law
- *Legislative Branch:* Enacts (votes to pass) the law
- *Judicial Branch:* Interprets and applies the law to disputes

Under the various federal and state constitutions in the United States, no branch is permitted to perform an essential function of another branch.

The Courts

Of course, the federal and various state constitutions do not specifically address every conflict that arises among people and companies. The legislature also cannot possibly write laws to cover each and every circumstance imaginable. For these reasons, a court system is needed to interpret and apply the law to the unique facts in the disputes that inevitably arise. In fulfilling its responsibility, the judiciary (often with a jury) hears carefully admitted, factual evidence.

Evidence. Often, a jury does not hear all the evidence. Some evidence may be considered "inadmissible" because of how it was obtained, because it is considered unfairly prejudicial, or because it is considered unreliable (e.g., hearsay). One exception to the general inadmissibility of hearsay is "records kept in the ordinary course of business" (e.g., incident reports and normal employee records documentation).

Appeals. After trial, a case may be **appealed** to a higher court, if one side thinks the trial judge erred in applying the law. Note: Facts found at trial usually cannot be appealed. If a case is appealed, judges then write **decisions** (also referred to as **opinions**) explaining how and why they interpreted and applied the law to a particular case. Opinions are then published and make up what is known as **case law (common law).**

Decisions. When hearing a case, the court first looks to see what written laws (i.e., statutes or rules and regulations) enacted by the legislature or by a responsible administrative agency exist. If no written law clearly decides the matter, the court looks to its own previous opinions—the common law it created. If the court decided a previous case one way, it will usually decide later cases the same way. Following past decisions is known as adhering to precedent. **Precedent** (also referred to as *stare decisis*) gives some predictability to the law. It helps all of us identify our obligations and rights under the law, even when our rights and responsibilities are not clearly spelled out by the legislature.

Administrative Agencies

To better respond to society's changing needs, both federal and state legislatures began establishing various "expert" regulatory bodies or agencies in the first part of this century. These agencies—such as the Equal Employment Opportunity Commission (EEOC), Department of Labor (DOL), Immigration and Naturalization Services (INS), Internal Revenue Service (IRS), National Labor Relations Board (NLRB), Occupational Safety and Health Administration (OSHA), and their sister agencies in state government—hold all the powers similar to those for each branch of government:

- *Legislative Power:* To establish rules and regulations that have the same effect as legislatively enacted laws
- *Executive Power:* To enforce the agency's rules by conducting investigations and inspections and by levying fines when an agency's rules are not followed
- *Judicial Power:* To hold hearings (similar to bringing a case to court) to decide whether an agency rule was in fact violated in a particular circumstance

To answer the questions posed at the beginning of this chapter—that is, to learn what law applies to a particular set of circumstances in our legal system—one must, in essence, do the following:

1. Determine whether the state or federal system has **jurisdiction** and which court or regulatory agency has authority
2. Determine whether the (federal or state) legislature has passed a law or whether an administrative agency has promulgated rules or regulations that apply
3. Review case law or administrative agency findings to see how the courts or administrative agencies interpreted and applied the law in similar cases

There is no simple answer to avoiding civil liability. There are, however, guidelines that apply. Being familiar with these guidelines can help you conduct yourself—and train and supervise others—in ways that minimize your risk and your institution's risk of being found liable for your action or inaction.

Civil Liability: Tort Law

Civil law in the United States is that vast collection of statutory and common law that deals with private rights and remedies. Although the state may be a party in civil law matters, the desired impact is to establish and adjudicate rights as between or among private persons, both natural and corporate.

One of the best ways to begin learning of the legal guidelines that affect you as a supervisor is to look at a very broad area of civil law known as torts. A **tort** is a willful or negligent wrong done to one person by another. Tort law encompasses most all aspects of the law, including statutory law, administrative rules and regulations, constitutional law, and common law.

Burden of Proof

At a civil trial, **plaintiffs** have the burden to prove each and every **element** of a civil case by a **preponderance of the evidence** (i.e., that all required elements are "more likely than not," or that they meet "more than a 50 percent" standard of certainty).

- *Criminal Court—Beyond a Reasonable Doubt:* In criminal court, the plaintiff must prove someone guilty "beyond a reasonable doubt," or by nearly 100%.
- *Civil Court—Preponderance of the Evidence:* In civil court, plaintiffs merely need to prove that the defendant's actions were incorrect by a 51% likelihood, or just a bit more than half the defendant's "burden."

Kinds of Torts

In general, there are two kinds of civilly actionable torts:

- Intentional
- Negligent

Intentional Torts. Intentional torts occur when someone acts *purposefully* and violates the legally protected rights of another. Intentional torts do not mean the responsible party *wanted to hurt* the plaintiff, only that the act was willful—and the resulting harm was *reasonably foreseeable*. The following are intentional torts:

- **Assault, battery**
- **Defamation**
- **False imprisonment (false arrest)**
- **Invasion of privacy**

Negligent Torts. Negligent torts occur when someone has a duty to act in a certain way and either *fails to act entirely or acts incompletely*. They are the result of a failure to use reasonable care and due diligence under the particular circumstances as a result of which another is injured or suffers some damage. **Negligence** does not require intent—even intent to be negligent. Rather, negligence is characterized by the absence of an attitude or intent to be duly careful.

To be negligent is to err. To err is simply human. Negligence is the stuff of everyday life in which people fail to do sensible things in ordinary situations. For example, a negligent tort may result from any of the following:

- Failure to report a burnt-out light
- Failure to properly clean up a spill in a corridor
- Failure to properly check identification at an access control point
- Failure to carefully monitor a prisoner patient
- Incomplete preliminary investigation of an unusual circumstance

The whole theory of negligence operates from the assumption that there is what is known as a reasonable person—an individual capable of adhering to a general standard of conduct. A reasonable person is not perfect or infallible. A reasonable person makes mistakes, but never are these mistakes gross or utterly careless. A reasonable person attempts to react intelligently and with valor during an emergency situation, but does not always reach that level. The reasonable person possesses generic knowledge about life, law, and the facts of the universe, but hardly could be characterized as an expert. In sum, the reasonable person is John and Jane Doe, and their lifestyles are the law's model human composition.

In the law of negligence, the reasonable person is the person who suffers. The unreasonable person is grossly careless, aggressive, and *carelessly* reactive and either does not have the necessary knowledge to function and exist properly in the world or chooses to disregard it. As a supervisor, you have an accepted standard of conduct; this standard is what guides your daily occupational habits and decision making.

Elements of a Tort

The term tort comes from the Latin word *torquere*, which means "to wrongfully twist aside." In a legal sense, the term tort describes situations where someone has a duty, but breaches it, which directly or indirectly causes damages. Taken apart, the four elements are these:

- ***Duty to Another:*** To act or not act
- ***Breach of Duty:*** Failure to fulfill the duty, either directly or indirectly
- ***Cause:*** Proximate or foreseeable
- ***Damage:*** To another person or the property of another person

Together, the four items make up the required elements of a tort. All elements must be found by a preponderance of the evidence in both intentional and negligent torts before liability can attach—to you or to your institution. Each element is discussed separately in the paragraphs that follow.

Duty

In general, there are three areas to look at when deciding what duty may exist in a particular case: laws, practices, and common sense.

Laws. A duty may be found under a **statute**, **rule** (regulation), or prior court **decision** that either requires or forbids certain actions.

Example 1: Both statutory and common law place a duty on all persons to avoid the *unprivileged* touching of (committing a battery upon) another person.

Example 2: Laws also prohibit us from falsely arresting another. In most jurisdictions, arrest is defined as restricting another's freedom of movement. No special words or actions are required.

Practices. A duty may be found in a security department's own rules and regulations, under a healthcare organization's policies and procedures, or even under common industry practice. Under any of these circumstances, a duty may exist even if such rules hold an officer to a higher standard of care than otherwise required by law.

Example: A security procedure states (or common practice by other security departments indicates) that officers conducting nighttime escorts should wait with the person being escorted until the person's car starts. A duty would then exist to wait until the car starts, even if no statute or case law requires the officer to do so.

Common Sense. A duty may also be found under a reasonable person (or common sense) standard, even if no law, security procedure, or common practice exists. In other words, what action would an ordinary person (not a security person) take or not take under similar circumstances?

Example: No law prohibits running in a hospital corridor. An officer, while responding to an alarm, ran into and knocked a patient off a stretcher. A duty not to run unreasonably fast in a hospital corridor may be found to exist under a reasonable person standard.

That the officer was responding to an emergency matters little. That the officer did not intend to hurt the patient also does not matter much. That security officers at other hospitals run in the corridors also likely does not matter.

Breach

A breach occurs when someone fails to fulfill a duty (either to act or not to act) in a manner proscribed by law, rule, regulation, prior court decision, common industry practice, self-imposed policy, or under the above reasonableness/common sense standard.

Cause

After proving a duty existed, that the defendant breached that duty, and that damages resulted, a plaintiff must also prove that the breach of duty was the cause of the damages that resulted. In general, there are two types of cause:

- Cause in fact
- Proximate (reasonably foreseeable) cause

Cause in Fact. Cause in fact exists where a defendant's actions were the "direct cause" of the plaintiff's injuries. In other words, "but for" the defendant's action (or inaction), the plaintiff would not have suffered the injury.

Example: An officer approached a trespasser in a hospital corridor, gave a verbal trespass warning, and ordered the person to leave the property. Instead of leaving, the trespasser began using foul language in a loud voice. In an attempt to quiet the trespasser, the officer drew his or her flashlight and warned the trespasser to leave or be forcibly removed. Upon further refusal of the trespasser to quiet down or leave the property, the officer struck the trespasser.

A jury will likely find that this officer had a duty not to use "unreasonable force" **(excessive force)**. The jury will likely also find that unreasonable force was used; as such, the officer breached his or her duty. Finally, the jury will likely find that the officer directly caused the resulting damages.

Proximate Cause. With proximate cause, on the other hand, a defendant's actions or "failure to act" make possible the foreseeable actions of another, such as a third-party criminal. In other words, as an "indirect result" of the defendant's inaction (the defendant being the officer or maybe you), a subsequent criminal act occurred that caused damage to the plaintiff.

Example: Unscheduled unlock and escort requests poured in one hectic evening. Your people were unable to get to their lockups at the scheduled times. Unbeknownst to anyone, a surgical supply salesperson forgot a $8500 laptop computer containing invaluable proprietary trade secret information in one of the executive conference rooms. The embarrassed salesperson returned at 8:25 p.m., walked in through an unlocked back door, and found the computer had been stolen. The salesperson and the surgical supply company sue you for breaching your duty to lock the doors on time and indirectly causing their damages.

Damages

Once it is determined that a duty existed, was breached, and caused damages, the next question is this: How and to what extent was the plaintiff harmed? Damages to a plaintiff range from very slight to extreme. Generally, three categories exist:

- Nominal damages
- Compensatory (actual) damages
- Punitive (exemplary) damages

Nominal Damages are very slight.

Compensatory (Actual) Damages exist where there is more than nominal injury to the plaintiff or the plaintiff's property. Compensatory damages are intended to make a victim whole. In other words, the intent is to financially compensate the victim for all losses resulting from the defendant's breach of duty.

Such compensation may, for example, include a monetary award for medical bills, pain and suffering, lost wages, loss of consortium, or replacement or repair of property.

Compensatory damages are also awarded where there has been an invasion of privacy, infliction of emotional distress, or damage to someone's reputation (i.e., **slander** or **libel**).

Punitive (Exemplary) Damages are awarded to punish a defendant for wrongful conduct as well as to send a message to others. State law determines when punitive damages may be awarded. In general, the defendant's conduct must be reckless, gross, wanton, or outrageous.

> *Example:* An officer escorted a woman to her car in the campus parking lot. Late for lunch, the officer left the woman before she started her car. The woman was then raped by a trespasser.
>
> A jury could find that, under security department policy (or by common security/industry practice), the officer had a duty to wait until the woman was safely proceeding out of the lot. Even without a security department policy (or law) to this effect, the jury could find a duty to wait with the woman under the reasonable person/common sense standard of duty, particularly in areas with high crime rates. Because there is no well-defined industry standard of a high crime area, this is a "question of fact" left to the jury, sometimes with the help of expert testimony. The jury might decide that the officer breached his duty by leaving. It appears that damages resulted. Finally, the jury might decide the officer's breach of duty was the proximate (foreseeable) cause of the woman's damages.
>
> Even though the officer did not participate in the rape and never intended that the woman be injured, leaving allowed a third party to commit the rape. This was a reasonably foreseeable consequence of the officer's action/inaction.

Vicarious Liability

After proving, by a preponderance of the evidence, that the four elements of a tort are present, the next question is, "Who is responsible for paying for the damages?" Obviously, the person who breached his or her duty can be required to pay. Others may also be found liable— even if they have not participated or were present at the time of the injury. Two such kinds of **vicarious liability** are discussed in the paragraphs that follow:

- *Respondeat superior*
- Negligent supervision

Respondeat Superior

The officer's employer(s) may be required to pay under a theory of law known as *respondeat superior*. Loosely translated, the Latin term means "the master answers for the acts of the servant." By vicarious liability, an employer, like a security supervisor or management team, having the right to govern, supervise, manipulate, and control the action of employees or agents, can be held accountable for an officer's actions. All that is required is that the officer was acting within the "scope of his or her employment" and not "off on a frolic." (Note: Many "off on a frolic" cases involve excessive force contrary to one's training and common sense.) Scope of employment is not narrowly defined. What is looked for is whether the officer's actions were directly or indirectly of *intended benefit* to the employer. Even if the benefit is slight, liability can attach.

Further, even if the officer's actions violated clearly established policies or procedures, this will not have much, if any, significance in reducing the employer's liability so long as the employee was acting within the scope of employment.

> *Example 1:* An off-duty officer visited a friend in one of the labs on campus. The officer suspected an individual of attempting to steal a microscope. Without further provocation or right to use "reasonable and necessary force" in self-defense, the officer struck the person on the back of the head.

Chapter 9: Civil Liability and the Supervisor

The officer's actions clearly violated procedure. Nevertheless, the organization may be liable, based on the doctrine of *respondeat superior*, as the officer's actions to prevent a theft were within the scope of employment.

Example 2: An officer was assigned to watch a patient at risk for elopement. The officer, deciding this activity was boring because the patient was sleeping and not going anywhere, headed upstairs to see a friend. The patient left, jumped a fence, and fell to her death.

This officer may be found to have been off on a frolic (i.e., pursuing his or her own self-interest) and, as such, "voided" the organization's liability insurance policy.

The status of the employer-employee relationship is fundamental to the question of eventual liability.

Duty to Properly Supervise

Another kind of vicarious liability may be found in cases where there is **negligent supervision** of an officer. Supervisors who fail to meet the required **standard of care** in supervising, training, counseling, or disciplining (including dismissal) subordinates may learn that not only can their institution be liable, but that they may be held "personally liable."

Example: An institution's fire insurance policy required that two watch-clock patrols be conducted in closed buildings each evening shift (duty). A fire occurred in one of the buildings late one evening shift (damages). On investigation, the insurance company learned the building in which the fire occurred was not patrolled on the evening in question, nor patrolled on most evenings over the past six months (breach and proximate cause).

The insurance company may decline to honor the insurance claim submitted. The company may also, if forced to pay the claim, sue the supervisors responsible for seeing that the watch-clock patrols were conducted (duty to supervise, breach, proximate cause, and damages).

In many jurisdictions, judgments are collectible for up to 20 years, possibly through the **garnishing** of wages, and are not dischargeable in bankruptcy.

A **cause of action** against a supervisor, as well as against an institution, may also exist as the result of other negligence, such as **negligent hiring, negligent retention,** or **negligent training.**

Negligent Hiring and Retention. The theory of negligent appointment or hiring has been litigated on occasion. Hiring an individual without investigating the person's background or improperly placing an individual in a position that requires higher levels of expertise than the applicant possesses are possible negligent appointments.

The courts have ruled that employees who have contact with members of the public (i.e., security officers) are held to an even higher standard of reasonable care in terms of hiring and retention. This requirement is imposed because it is reasonably foreseeable that such an employee could cause an unreasonable risk of injury to the public. Simply put, a security supervisor who appoints or hires security officers to perform specific tasks must know or should know that their appointments are competent to carry out their jobs.

When a supervisor knows, and should know, that an employee is inept and dismissible, but chooses instead to take no action, a judgment of negligent retention is possible. Negligent retention is the breach of an employer's duty to be aware of an employee's unfitness and to take corrective action through retraining, reassignment, or discharge. Care must be taken when the responsibilities of an employee are changed over a period of time.

While implementing a dismissal or termination of any employee is a difficult task, case law and common sense dictate that retaining an employee who has been and will continue to be troublesome will cause longer term difficulties. Pre-employment testing and evaluations, post-employment training and evaluation, and adequate supervision corresponding to carefully drafted guidelines and policies are protective shields. Failure to take these minimal precautions may leave the supervisor facing liability unnecessarily.

Negligent Supervision and Training. Once an employee is hired and assigned, as a supervisor you have a continuing obligation to exercise a duty of due care relative to employee operations. The vast majority of cases related to security involve the action or inaction of security officers and the failure to supervise them properly. A failure to supervise or manage can be the supervisor's failure to hire sufficient personnel, to insufficiently or improperly train shift supervisors or other secondary managerial employees, or to allot sufficient time and energy to train employees for appropriate tasks. This includes having an appropriate employee knowledge verification system.

The final theory under the negligence umbrella is negligent training. The bottom line is your security officers must be adequately trained. Moreover, the training they receive must be sufficiently practical to enable them to demonstrate technical and legal competency commensurate with the duties they perform. Classroom theory is not enough. Academics should be combined with performance exercises so that officers can practice and become confident with the techniques they may be required to use.

Legal Issues in Managing Employees

Twenty-five years ago, relatively few pieces of legislation affected the employer-employee relationship. Since then, major employment laws have increased ten-fold, with no slowdown in sight. Further, the courts have become more receptive to enforcing common law employment lawsuits. The majority of problems employers face are concentrated in a few areas and quite common to healthcare and the security industry.

As noted earlier, laws are constantly changing to meet society's evolving needs and expectations. Although startling news to some, the most regulated and litigated aspect of any business today is said to be in employment matters.

Employment at Will

As recently as the 1950s, employees had few rights with respect to their employment. Relatively few state and federal laws affected employment relationships, and there were even fewer court decisions on the topic. Absent a written contract, employment relationships were governed by the doctrine of "at-will employment." At-will employment gave employees and employers the right to end the employment relationship at any time, with or without cause and with or without notice.

Today, employees have many rights with respect to their employment. Currently, approximately 80 federal laws impact employment relationships and many more state laws. Over time, judges and juries that continue to carve out exceptions to it, while still in existence, have significantly eroded the doctrine of at-will employment.

In most healthcare security departments, employees are hired "at will." This is interpreted to mean that the employer hires an individual for an indefinite period of time and either party may terminate the relationship without cause or notice. However, there are exceptions to this broad rule. Do not presume at-will employment is absolute; it can be rebutted under certain circumstances.

Wrongful Discharge. When reviewing the exceptions to employment at will, the theory of "wrongful discharge" comes into consideration. Wrongful discharge describes an employment termination that violates common law principles or statutory law. Wrongful discharge cases can be categorized into three general types:

- Public policy violations
- Breach of an implied contract
- Tort claims

Public policy means the rights of one person are limited by the rights of others and the public. Certain actions by an employer and by you as a supervisor are therefore prohibited. Numerous **acts** (laws) prohibit discharge of an employee based on illegal discrimination or retaliation for exercising rights under the law. For example, the Age Discrimination in Employment Act, Americans with Disabilities Act, Equal Pay Act of 1963, Title

VII of Civil Rights Act of 1964, Family and Medical Leave Act, and the Uniform Services Employment and Reemployment Rights Act are a few. The following are examples of where a discharge might violate public policy:

- Employee refuses to violate the law as part of his or her work duties
- Employee "blows the whistle" on the employer's illegal, unsafe, or improper practices
- Employee exercises a specific statutory right or privilege (e.g., recently filed a Workers' Compensation claim, testified as a witness against the company, engaged in union activities)

Avoiding Legal Action by Employees
Employment contracts typically address length, terms, and conditions of employment. They can, however, be complicated to interpret as the parties to the contract may or may not apply the employment-at-will doctrine. Most employees do *not* work under a written employment contract, but an employment contract may be implied from written documents (offer letters, handbooks, and so on), verbal remarks (job interview assurances, management promises and commitments), or company practices.

All supervisors should understand that even if your organization does everything lawfully, you still can be sued for wrongful conduct. Employers who do things that are unfair or bizarre may be held liable even if there is no prior law on the subject. Courts may broaden an existing law or apply a rule retroactively.

So how do you prepare for such uncertainty? To best understand, put on your employee hat and look at what employees want from their supervisor and employer. As the sidebar shows, the things employees want are quite simplistic.

What Employees Want
- To see clear, understandable, and publicized rules or policies
- To hear performance expectations
- To receive frank feedback on performance and conduct
- To be treated uniformly in the application of company standards and work rules
- To receive a thorough investigation of allegations of misconduct
- To tell their side of the story
- To be apprised of an investigation's outcome
- To receive warning before discharge
- To use a process of review by management other than their direct supervisor

When making decisions that impact the employer-employee relationship, consider how the decision will affect the workplace: How will it affect employee relations? What will your employees think and how will they respond?

All these factors contribute to making good documentation by supervisors and managers an essential part of contemporary work relationships.

Role of Good Documentation Regarding Employees

Documentation is often important for reasons no one could have foreseen. That is why supervisors and managers must document incidents of both greater and lesser significance, even without knowing how the documentation may one day be used. In a legal dispute, good documentation of the events leading up to or surrounding the discipline or discharge can be a crucial part of the employer's proof that the decision was good and reasonable.

> **Ways Documentation Helps the Supervisor and Employer**
> - Proof in lawsuits and charges filed with administrative agencies
> - Improve employee morale, productivity, and efficiency
> - Proof in administrative hearings (unemployment)
> - Support for discharge or other disciplinary action
> - Reminders at time of performance appraisals

Standards for Both Sides

In the employee's eyes, the reasons for a disciplinary action or discharge may be anything but good and reasonable. However, courts and administrative agencies have upheld the employer's (supervisor's) ability to establish standards for employee behavior and performance and to discipline and discharge anyone who fails to meet those standards, even if the judge or jury might have set different standards.

Realize, however, that in setting standards the employer is suggesting to employees that if they meet those standards they can be reasonably assured of keeping their jobs. Thus, the employer must base any judgments about performance or continued employment on the standards that have been clearly expressed. This means the employer is held to the standard of not suddenly and arbitrarily changing the rules. The employer may have to demonstrate that it acted in good faith.

Role of Disciplinary Process

Progressive discipline is a well-established employee relations system. A progressive disciplinary process enables you to do the following:
- Apply standards or job objectives
- Judge your employees against the established standards or objectives
- Except in serious cases of misconduct, take progressively more serious steps in the disciplinary process until the employee improves, resigns, or is discharged

Value of Documentation on Employees
- Creates a history
- Aids memory
- Reveals patterns or changes in patterns (i.e., yo-yo behavior)
- Allows analysis and makes concrete the employer's thoughts and concerns
- Encourages continuation of positive behaviors
- Causes behavior modification of negative behavior
- Lends credibility to employer version of events
- Proves the employer's case in a trial, hearing, or arbitration
- Investigating

Should there be a legal dispute over your employment action, documentation of the steps you have taken in the disciplinary process can help you in several ways:
- Demonstrate that you did not act suddenly or arbitrarily; demonstrate that you conducted a long-term effort to raise the employee's performance up to expected standards
- Demonstrate that you made a constructive effort to improve the employee's performance and that discharge was a legitimate last resort
- Effectively rebut any claims by the employee that he or she was never told of the requirement

- Offset the less favorable evidence on the record, such as a history of ignoring other violations or a succession of good evaluations in the personnel file

Always remember that while progressive discipline is encouraged, it may not be necessary or even appropriate in every circumstance. If, in the opinion of the employer, a violation of work rules or an incident of inappropriate behavior is serious enough, any and all steps in the disciplinary process may be taken, up to and including discharge.

In a legal dispute, documentation of the disciplinary process provides powerful evidence for the employer. It shows the employer acted *reasonably* and the employee was treated *fairly*. In all but the most serious cases, courts and agencies like to see that an employee was given warnings followed by opportunities to improve performance or behavior before being discharged.

Remember, *the overall purpose of good documentation and discipline is to bring about a change in behavior or an improvement in employee performance.* The purpose is never to punish, humiliate, or otherwise embarrass the employee, but rather to correct inadequate performance or inappropriate behavior. Good documentation is the proof that you acted reasonably and that the employee was treated fairly and not disciplined or discharged for an illegal reason. You must document the steps you take. By directing the documentation to the employee and ensuring he or she has a copy, you are demonstrating your good faith effort to help the employee take corrective action necessary to successfully improve performance or stop problem behavior.

As a supervisor, you need to remember to document both good and bad performance and behavior. Many supervisors tend to only document those incidents that result in discipline. Instead, supervisors should keep ongoing notes of both the good and bad things employees do. This enables you to better recognize patterns of behavior that may need to be addressed at a later date. Also, documenting the good things employees do can be just as important as documenting the bad. Employees appreciate positive feedback and deserve to be rewarded for their hard work.

To ensure accuracy, documentation should be done as close in time to the performance or behavior as possible. If the incident results in discipline, the disciplinary action itself should also be taken as close in time to the performance or behavior as possible. A lag between the performance or behavior and the resulting documentation and/or disciplinary action may subject the documentation or action to greater challenge in a legal dispute.

Nothing in the personnel file should be a surprise to the employee. Documentation of behavior or performance problems should be discussed with and, ideally, signed by the employee before being placed in the personnel file.

The Supervisor's Log

In addition to putting documentation in the personnel file, every supervisor should keep a running log that records the behavior and performance of employees. Decide where you can access and maintain this log most conveniently, yet privately. You may find it best to keep your log in a daily planner, calendar, diary, notebook, or computer file. Entries should contain a brief summary of the important facts that you can use to refresh your memory. These notes need not be a verbatim rendition of the entire incident or conversation. Entries into the log should include information such as the following:

- Job performance
- On-the-job behavior
- Performance objectives
- Training
- Counseling
- Tardiness and absenteeism
- Discipline

Do not make entries that you would not want to be discovered in a legal dispute, as entries made are discoverable in litigation.

Discrimination

Everyone discriminates in one way or another. Some people prefer a blue sedan to a red convertible; others prefer steak to chicken; and most supervisors want to hire, retain, groom, and promote the best, most deserving person. All of the above is legal.

Liability for *illegal* **discrimination** occurs when one makes (or even seems to have a predisposition to make) job-related decisions based on the following:[1]

- Age
- Race
- National origin
- Religion
- Gender
- Marital status
- Veteran status
- Physical disability
- Sexual orientation (in some jurisdictions)

Persons within the above "protected classes" have for years received the enhanced judicial protection of "close scrutiny" when they present a *prima facie* case of different/disparate treatment in the workplace and elsewhere. The "burden of proof" can then shift to the defendant to prove the reasons for treating others differently were not a "pretext" to excuse the defendant's illegal discriminatory actions.

As such, you must do your best to avoid even the appearance of impropriety or unfairness by consistently doing the following with all your staff: (1) applying all policies and procedures, (2) assigning all work and work schedules, and (3) offering opportunities to learn and grow.

The need for consistency and fairness exists not only in the downside of taking disciplinary or corrective counseling action (including, but not limited to termination), but also in the upside of bestowing opportunities, raises, assignments, and other personnel actions.

Do not confuse illegal discrimination with a lowering of work standards or relaxed performance expectations. You can continue to maintain high standards within your department or institution if your supervisory team enforces its standards and rewards all your people fairly and consistently.

Sexual Harassment

For a number of years, and in most jurisdictions, the definition of sexual harassment was limited to situations where *sexual favors were sought, even indirectly, by a supervisor with only an implied promise of favorable treatment* (e.g. promotion, raise, assignment, days off) in return.

Today, many courts have expanded the definition of sexual harassment to prohibit "hostile work environments." A hostile environment can be found when on-the-job behavior (or even an off-the-job act such as at an informal gathering of employees) is such that a reasonable man or woman would consider such behavior offensive. The *quid pro quo* of a sexual favor is *no longer* a required element.

Sexually oriented jokes and cartoons, assignments based on sex, or even passing comments about one's own or another's sexual experiences can all be used as evidence to show a hostile environment existed.

Some legislatures are now following the court's lead and enacting laws governing the definition of sexual harassment, a hostile environment, and so on.

In many jurisdictions, the court need not be shown that a supervisor engaged in offensive behavior—only that, by a preponderance of evidence, a supervisor should have known such behavior was engaged in by others and took no real steps to stop it.

---

[1] Except, possibly, a disability that significantly hinders job performance (e.g., "places the safety of others in danger") and for which no "reasonable accommodation" can be made.

Example: A female officer was hired. She overheard a mild sexual joke and topped it with a raunchier one. She went on to tell even coarser jokes to others and gained a reputation as one of the best joke-tellers in the department. Not only that, she swore profusely and told frequent stories about her own sexual exploits.

This officer was later passed over for a promotion she felt she deserved (but did not) and sued for being forced to work in a hostile environment.

You defended yourself, claiming that the jokes and other sexually related antics were her doing. She, in turn, testified that to be accepted, she felt she needed to... and that "while my supervisor cautioned me a few times, he never made me stop."

Admittedly, under most states' current law, she would not prevail under the above facts. But remember this: the idea is not just to win, but to avoid becoming a defendant in the first place. Under our system, the costs of defending one's self are not only considerable, but usually not recoverable from the other side—even if you do win. As is sometimes said: even when you win in court, you lose.

Americans with Disabilities Act of 1990

Of all the federal laws that influence how you hire and manage workers, the most complicated and demanding is the Americans with Disabilities Act (ADA). The ADA, which went into full effect in July 1994, provides employment and other protections to an estimated 43 million Americans with physical or mental disabilities. This law requires public accommodations be made accessible and that public entities and utilities provide needed services for disabled people.

Title I of the ADA deals with how employers deal with disabled workers and job applicants. The law forbids employers from discriminating on the basis of disability in hiring, promoting, or compensating workers. It requires employers to make "reasonable accommodations" for disabled workers who can otherwise perform the essential functions of a job. Its protection also extends to people currently well but with a history of disability, people wrongly perceived as having a disability and—to a limited extent—people related to individuals with a disability.

The law's definition of disability is vague and subject to much judicial interpretation. The ADA says that a disabled worker must inform his or her employer of any disability that requires accommodation. Because the ADA is complicated and vague at the same time, as a supervisor, you must know and understand your organization's policies as well as understand the importance of maintaining a diverse and qualified workforce.

The Process of a Civil Suit

Complaint
Lawsuits begin with a set of facts set out by a plaintiff (i.e., a party alleging injury) in a **complaint** filed with the court, which generally describes the facts, the duty breached, and the damages suffered. As part of their strategy, many plaintiffs name as many defendants as possible. Two primary reasons for this are (1) they hope at least one will be found liable, and (2) they hope a defendant will help the plaintiff's case by blaming another defendant for the damages.

Answer
The alleged wrongdoers (the defendants) then file an **answer** to the complaint, which either denies certain facts or the law relied on by the plaintiff or explains why the defendants were legally justified in taking the action in the complaint.

The defendant may also counter-sue the plaintiff.

Discovery
A pretrial process known as **discovery** then begins. Both parties use the discovery process to learn about the other's case. Discovery includes the taking of sworn **depositions,** the submission of **interrogatories** (sending written questions to the other party), and the serving of **subpoena** *duces tecum* (requiring the other party to provide copies of documents—many of which often seem irrelevant).

Report Writing. We have all heard of the need for well-written factual reports. Such reports are used for investigative purposes and for compiling statistics. They are also discoverable (able to be obtained) by parties to a suit.

Hunches, conclusions, opinions, excuses, and so on contained in a report frequently are used against the report writer and the employer in the event of a suit. If a report is in improper form for any of the above reasons, the time to correct it is *before* it has been accepted by the supervisor.

When writing a report that includes "facts" that you or your officer do not personally know to be true, *cite* (name) your *source* of information. And, where possible and relevant, *quote* the person who provided the information. Never divulge confidential information outside the department.

Trial

If a case is not settled during the discovery process, the case then proceeds to trial. Either party may insist upon a "trial by jury." A jury's role is to hear evidence and make "findings of fact" by a "preponderance of the evidence." If a case is heard without a jury, the judge makes the findings of fact. The judge makes rulings of law throughout the case (e.g., what evidence is discoverable, admissible).

Appeal

After a decision is reached, either party may ask a higher court to review the decision (i.e., appeal). An appeal must be based on an alleged error in applying the law and usually may not be based on a dispute over what facts have been found.

How Not to Become a Defendant

There are steps that you as a supervisor and your organization need to take to avoid becoming a defendant or, at minimum, to help defend yourself and/or your institution in the event of a lawsuit. These steps apply whether you are accused of providing negligent security or of violating a provision of the state employment law. In essence, you must do the following:

- Take responsibility
- Be consistent, cautious, open, and fair
- Use all the tools available to you

Details on each of these are presented in the paragraphs that follow.

Take Responsibility

Supervisors are held to a higher standard because they are representatives of their institution's administrations. Know this and provide your people with leadership by example. Model the way and set a high mark. Do not rely on "finger pointing." Do not believe that you will escape liability because you did not know or were only following orders.

Be Consistent, Cautious, Open, and Fair

Track your own actions to be consistent in what you do. Do not be defensive; instead, learn from your mistakes and be responsive to those supervised. Give all employees "due process," by being available and open to listening. Investigate thoroughly and then decide.

Use All Tools Available to You

Ask for the help and guidance of your own manager and fellow supervisors. Do not sleepwalk through the performance review process. Be advised that many suits related to employment law are lost because of a supervisor's past unwillingness to "step up" and fairly "mark down" someone's substandard performance.

Key Terms

Act: Legislative act, also known as law or statute. When pending, an act is known as a bill. When passed (i.e., enacted), a bill is referred to as a law, statute, or act.

Action: Also known as legal action, lawsuit, or criminal action. Refers to entire process where one party moves against another party in an effort to obtain damages, require specific performance, or obtain criminal conviction, etc. *See also Cause of Action.*

Answer: Defendant's written response to a plaintiff's complaint.

Appeal: Resort to a higher court to challenge the decision of an inferior court or administrative agency. Generally, appeals may only challenge interpretations of the law and may not challenge findings of fact.

Assault: Intentional (willful) attempt or threat to inflict injury upon another coupled with the apparent present ability to do so. (A completed offensive touching is not a required element.)

Battery: A completed offensive touching of another without justification or excuse.

Bill: *See Act.*

Case Law: *See Common Law.*

Cause of Action: The facts that give someone the legal right to judicial relief (i.e., to recover damages).

Common Law: Also known as case law and distinguished from an act of the legislature; includes all judgments and decrees of the court interpreting and applying acts of the legislature and recognizing common custom and usage, especially the ancient unwritten law of England.

Complaint: The original writing (initial pleading) filed by a plaintiff with a court commencing (beginning) an action. Complaints must allege facts, which state a sufficiently legal cause of action.

Decision: *See Opinion.*

Defamation: Includes both libel (the written word you can look at) and slander (the spoken word). Communication that is false and tends to injure the reputation of another; untrue communication that ridicules another.

Defendant: The party against whom a law suit is brought (i.e., the alleged wrongdoer, the wrongdoer's supervisor, the wrongdoer's employer, etc.).

Deposition: *See Discovery.*

Discovery: Pretrial means that can be used by parties to an action and that enable the parties to learn about the facts of the other party's case. Devices include deposition (i.e., sworn testimony under oath in front of an authorized court officer, usually occurring in an attorney's office), interrogatories (i.e., written questions requiring written responses from the other party), and subpoena *duces tecum* (i.e., the other party must produce copies of documents related to a case).

Discrimination: Treatment of another that is not consistent with others whether with regard to disciplinary action or rewards.

Duty of Care: Employers have a duty to exercise reasonable care in hiring individuals who, because of the type of employment and amount of contact with the public, may pose a threat of injury to members of the public.

Elements: The separate parts of a cause of action (or crime) that must be proven (e.g., duty, breach, damages, and cause are the elements of a tort).

Excessive Force: The use of force beyond that which is "reasonable and necessary" to complete a legal act. In many jurisdictions, excessive force by a private citizen is any force beyond that necessary to effect a "retreat" from the danger posed by another.

False Imprisonment (False Arrest): Unlawful restriction on an individual's freedom of movement. (Malice is not a required element and no specific words are required.)

Garnish: A legal order where an employer is required by the court to withhold and forward monies from a defendant's pay.

Inadequate Security: Security measures provided to safeguard employees, customers, and members of the public that were not consistent with the potential threat.

Intent (also intentional): In legal usage, usually refers to purposeful action. Usually, there is no need for proof of an intended result, as long as the act in and of itself was intentional as distinguished from accidental or negligent.

Interrogatories: *See Discovery.*

Invasion of Privacy: The making public of facts to which one has a legally enforceable expectation of privacy. Unlike defamation, truth is not an available defense in a privacy action. Eavesdropping, making public security department or patient records, wire taps, or surreptitious audio or video surveillance may constitute invasion of privacy depending on applicable state and federal law.

Jurisdiction: Authority to act within a specific area. Can refer to geographic area (e.g., a state police officer has power to act—jurisdiction—as a police officer throughout the state). Also can refer to area of authority (e.g., probate court has jurisdiction over divorce cases and wills, but has no jurisdiction over criminal matters).

Libel: *See Defamation.*

Negligence: The omission or commission of something that an ordinary, reasonable, and prudent person would or would not do under similar circumstances.

Negligent Hiring: Failing to properly screen employees, resulting in the hiring of someone with a history of violent or criminal acts.

Negligent Retention: Retaining an employee after the employer became aware of the employee's unsuitability, thereby failing to act on that knowledge.

Negligent Supervision: Failing to provide the necessary monitoring to ensure that employees perform their duties properly.

Opinion: Statement written by a judge(s) explaining why a case was decided in a particular way; sometimes referred to as a decision. *See also Common Law and Precedent.*

Preponderance of the Evidence: The standard of proof used in a civil case whereby the plaintiff shows a fact to be "more likely than not" (i.e., more than a 50 percent certainty). Distinguished from proof "beyond a reasonable doubt," which is used in criminal cases.

Plaintiff: The party who starts (i.e., brings) a civil action against another to seek relief (e.g., for monetary damages or an order for specific performance).

Precedent: A case previously decided by the court that is similar to the facts and legal issues found in the case at hand and that therefore gives the court guidance in deciding the present case. Also referred to as *stare decisis*.

Respondeat Superior: A kind of vicarious liability. Latin for "let the master answer." Means an employer will be held responsible for certain actions of the employee. Also means a principal can be held to answer for acts of its agent.

Rule: Also known as regulation. Standard or guide established by authority empowered by legislature. Accorded same effect as legislatively enacted law.

Sexual Harassment: "Settled law" is any direct or implied request for sexual favors that may result in preferential treatment. "Emerging law" is any sexually "hostile environment" "allowed to exist," whether or not directly engaged in or encouraged by a supervisor.

Slander: *See Defamation.*

Standard of Care: The degree of care that should be exercised under a particular set of circumstances. The standard required may be found at law or under a reasonably prudent, ordinary person test.

Stare Decisis: See Precedent.

Statute: *See Act.*

Subpoena *Duces Tecum: See Discovery.*

Summons: Writing given by a court to a sheriff, or other official, for service upon (delivery to) a person notifying such person that an action has been filed against him/her/it in court.

Tort: Violations of a duty or other wrong for which an injured party may seek judicial relief.

Vicarious Liability: *See* Respondeat Superior.

Bibliography

Michael, K. Esq. and J. F. Vaughan. 2003. *Avoiding Liability in Hospital Security*, 2nd ed. Atlanta: Strafford Publication Inc.

Mountain States Employers Council, Inc. 2002. Legal Issues in Managing Employees (presentation).

Mountain States Employers Council, Inc. 2002. The Role of Good Documentation (presentation).

Nemeth, C. P. 2005. *Private Security and the Law*, 3rd ed. Burlington, Mass: Elsevier Butterworth-Heinemann.

Williams, T. L. (ed.). 2007. *Protection of Assets*. Vol. 11. Los Angeles: ASIS International.

Study and Review Questions

1. A cause of negligent action against a supervisor, as well as against an institution, may be found in which of these?

    A. Hiring

    B. Retention

    C. Training

    D. All of the above

2. What are the four elements that must always be proven in a tort action?

    A. Duty, breach, cause, and damages

    B. Duty, expectation, cause, and concern

    C. Duty, violation, reason, and damages

    D. None of the above

3. What is the burden of proof a plaintiff must show in a tort case against a supervisor or an institution?

    A. Beyond a reasonable doubt

    B. By a preponderance of the evidence

    C. By conviction by a jury of peers

    D. All of the above

4. For what reason should a supervisor document employee performance?

    A. To protect the supervisor in the event of civil action

    B. To punish an employee for inadequate performance or inappropriate behavior

    C. To bring about a change in behavior or an improvement in employee performance

    D. To create a history that is shared with other employees to learn from the mistake

5. Sexual harassment is defined as what?
    A. Asking for sexual favors
    B. Sharing sexually oriented jokes and cartoons
    C. Giving out work assignments based on sex
    D. All of the above

Chapter 10

Safety and the Supervisor's Responsibilities

Tracy L. Buchman, MS, CHSP, CHPA

OBJECTIVES

After studying this chapter, the student should understand the following:

- The supervisor's responsibilities in protecting staff and customers in the healthcare environment
- The external organizations—regulatory, accrediting, and advisory—that collaborate with the healthcare institution to maintain a safe environment
- The objectives of the Safety Management program
- Specific hazards in the healthcare environment and precautions appropriate for security officers' personal safety
- Risks associated with magnetic resonance imaging (MRI) and precautions appropriate for security officers' personal safety

Healthcare is a unique setting for security work. The security supervisor is challenged with managing the safety of the customer served and the security officer.

Unique hazards are present in this environment. The stresses of coping with illness and injury can lead patients and visitors to act out. In interactions with patients and others, security officers may be exposed to blood-borne diseases (viruses such as hepatitis B and C and human immunodeficiency virus) and other transmissible pathogens. These are not uncommon in the healthcare environment. Another hazard is the potential for you and your security staff to receive harmful exposure to magnetic fields and the many chemicals used by ancillary departments.

Ensuring that officers follow safety guidelines is your responsibility. As a security supervisor, you must be familiar with the regulatory and accrediting agencies your institution collaborates with to maintain a safe environment for staff, patients, and visitors. You not only must be able to recognize specific hazards that are present in the environment in which you and your security staff work, you also must be able to quickly recognize the safety precautions that should be taken when working around them. Whenever the safety of others is in question, you must exercise your authority to make decisions. The basics for protecting your own safety and the safety of your security officers are the focus of this chapter.

External Organizations

Regulatory and advisory agencies influence the overall accreditation of the healthcare organization. As a security supervisor, you should be familiar with the mission of each of the following external organizations as it relates to security issues:

- *The Joint Commission:* According to the Joint Commission Web site, this organization's mission is "to continuously improve the safety and quality of care provided to the public through the provision of health care accreditation and related services that support performance improvement in health care organizations"

- *Occupational Safety and Health Administration (OSHA):* According to the OSHA Web site, this organization's mission is "to assure the safety and health of America's workers by setting and enforcing standards; providing training, outreach, and education; establishing partnerships; and encouraging continual improvement in workplace safety and health"
- *Centers for Disease Control and Prevention (CDC):* The CDC Web site states this organization's mission as "to promote health and quality of life by preventing and controlling disease, injury, and disability"

Safety Management

The Joint Commission views the Safety Management plan as the foundation of your organization's safety program. Regulations set by the OSHA Standards for General Industry (29 CFR Part 1910) and The Joint Commission are the foundation for the Safety Management plan.

Twice each year, your institution must conduct a hazard surveillance of all patient care areas. Each year, a Hazard Vulnerability Analysis (HVA) must be conducted. The HVA examines the impact of buildings, grounds, equipment, occupants, and internal physical systems on patient and public safety. The HVA is a continuous process, and the document gets updated as changes occur.

The security officer and security supervisor act as ambassadors for the organization and often participate in these assessments during patrols. Once issues are found and identified, requests for correction are completed. The security supervisor and officers evaluate the status of corrections during ongoing patrols.

The Safety Management program has the following objectives:

- To minimize accidents and injuries to patients, staff, visitors, and students
- To reduce or control costs for Workers' Compensation and costs associated with liability and litigation of patient and visitor incidents
- To assist in documentation of compliance for the OSHA and other regulatory agents
- To identify opportunities for improving performance, with the overall goal of improving total quality
- To manage how changes are implemented and track their success
- To keep abreast of changes in the healthcare industry
- To participate in the institution's plans for continuous improvement of work processes

Safety Hazards Common in the Healthcare Environment

As a security supervisor, you must ensure that your security staff are aware of the variety of safety hazards present in the environment in which they work. Ensure your staff members have been appropriately trained and that they apply their training consistently in their work. Working in healthcare settings, security personnel must be especially alert to three types of hazards:

- Serious infectious diseases
- Strong magnets
- Toxic chemicals

Appropriate precautions for working around each of these types of hazards are discussed separately below.

Following Standard Precautions for Infection Control

Managing uncooperative patients is a common task for security personnel. This work exposes you and your staff to a variety of hazards, including blood and other body fluids. Contact with these fluids can expose you and your security staff to infectious diseases.

The CDC has developed a set of standard precautions for infection control in healthcare personnel (www.cdc.gov/ncidod/dhqp/gl_hcpersonnel.html) and for isolation precautions in hospitals (www.cdc.gov/ncidod/dhqp/gl_isolation.html). These guidelines help protect healthcare workers from acquiring a patient's infection or spreading infection among patients. These standard precautions, summarized in the sidebar, describe how to deal with the following patient materials and body sites:

- Blood
- Secretions
- Skin that is not intact
- Body fluids
- Excretions, excluding sweat
- Mucous membranes

Remember, you and your security staff must routinely and consistently use standard precautions to reduce your risk of acquiring an infection from a patient or of inadvertently spreading infection among patients. The following are simple "rules of thumb" to which you and your security staff should always adhere:

- *If it is wet and human:* Do not touch it without gloves.
- *If it is wet and human, and it may splash or spray:* Protect your mucous membranes (particularly nostrils, lips, and ears) and skin.
- *If it is sharp:* Use safety-designed alternatives (after proper training). Use with utmost caution. Dispose of these items in a sharps container *immediately* after use.

Standard Precautions

Ensure your staff members know and use the following standard precautions. Provide regular training and refresher training to ensure your personnel's safety and compliance.

- *Avoid needle-sticks* and other injuries from sharp medical instruments: Use all sharp items carefully. Make use of available safety devices. Dispose of all such items immediately. Do not recap needles (see the bloodborne pathogens section in this chapter).

- *Wear gloves* when touching blood, body fluids, secretions, excretions, and contaminated items. Put on clean gloves just before touching a patient's mucous membranes and non-intact skin.

- *Perform hand hygiene* after touching blood, body fluids, secretions, excretions, and contaminated items, whether or not you wore gloves.

- *Wear a mask and eye protection or a face shield* during procedures likely to generate splashes or sprays of blood, body fluids, secretions, or excretions. This protects the mucosa (moist areas) of your eyes, nose, and mouth.

- *Wear a gown* during procedures likely to generate splashes or sprays of blood, body fluids, secretions, or excretions. This protects your skin and clothing.

- *Carefully handle* used patient care equipment in a manner that prevents skin and mucous membrane exposures, contamination of clothing, and transfer of microorganisms to other patients and environments. The equipment may be soiled with blood, body fluids, secretions, and excretions.

Important! You and your security staff must use standard precautions with *all patients* and *all moist body substances* (except sweat) at *all times*—regardless of the patient's age, gender, lifestyle, or diagnosis or whether the patient is under isolation for a specific disease.

Avoiding Blood-borne Pathogens

Blood-borne pathogens include HIV (human immunodeficiency virus), HBV (hepatitis B virus), and HCV (hepatitis C virus). Viruses such as these can be spread by contact with blood or other body fluids. Strictly following standard precautions—especially the precautions aimed at avoiding injuries from "sharps"—is essential to minimize the risk of acquiring these infections in the healthcare setting. Symptoms of HIV, HBV, and HCV infection are summarized below.

HBV and HCV. Both of these viruses cause hepatitis (inflammation of the liver). Symptoms of either infection typically develop slowly and may include fatigue, loss of appetite, generalized abdominal discomfort, nausea, and vomiting. The skin or the whites of the eyes may also become yellow (jaundice). About 30 percent of persons infected with hepatitis B virus and 80 percent of those infected with hepatitis C virus will have *no recognized symptoms*.

HIV. An infection with HIV sometimes results in a generalized mononucleosis-like illness that occurs several weeks or months after initial infection. Symptoms may include fever, sore throat, body aches, swollen lymph nodes, and rash. Up to 50 percent of persons recently infected with HIV will have *no recognized symptoms*. After this initial mild illness, the individual may not experience any symptoms related to HIV infection for months or years, until increasing damage to the immune system results in secondary infections or cancers.

Safety Around MRI Equipment

Many medical facilities have magnetic resonance imaging (MRI) equipment. Most MRI systems contain a 1.5-T magnet, which is very powerful and has approximately 30,000 times the magnetic pull of the earth. Some MRI magnets are even stronger than this. MRI equipment also uses radio frequency pulses. MRI is safe to the human body since it uses natural forces already in nature. The most important concept to remember in MRI safety is this:

- ***The magnet is always on!*** It is *never* off. It is *always* a magnet.

Many organizations have a proactive marking system to identify those objects that are "MRI SAFE." These are usually marked with a green sticker. Often, objects that are not MRI compatible are indicated with a red sticker marked as "NOT MRI SAFE."

MRI Safe Practice Guidelines

The importance of safety considerations has grown as MRI systems and technology improved. The static magnetic field generated by MRI systems attracts ferromagnetic objects with considerable force. Recent articles in the medical literature and electronic and print media have summarized adverse incidents involving patients, equipment, and personnel. The increasing popularity of stronger (3-T) systems have prompted experts to develop MRI Safe Practice Guidelines. These guidelines identify zones in the MRI suite and surrounding rooms.

Designating these zones has considerably decreased the incidence of adverse events. The MRI site is conceptually divided into four zones.

- ***Zone I:*** This includes all areas that are freely accessible to the public.
- ***Zone II:*** This is the interface between the publicly accessible, uncontrolled zone I and the strictly controlled zones III and IV.
- ***Zone III:*** Zone III regions should be physically restricted from general public access. A reliable, physically restricting method, such as access control, can differentiate between MRI personnel and non-MRI personnel.

- **Zone IV:** This is the MRI magnet room itself. As part of zone IV site restriction, all MRI installations should enable direct visual observation by zone II MRI personnel to access pathways into zone IV regions. The MRI technologists should be able to directly observe and control the entrances or access corridors to zone IV regions from their normal positions when stationed at their desks in the scan control room.

Of utmost importance, you and your security staff must understand basic safety so that you can safely enter the magnet room if need be or prevent others from entering a hazardous situation. People must not enter the scan room if they have any of the following:

- Pacemaker
- Aneurysm clips in the brain
- Neurostimulators
- Any other implants that have not been checked for safety by an MRI technologist

An MRI magnet erases all magnetically stored information. Thus, an MRI system renders the following items useless:

- Credit and bank cards
- Film
- Computer disks

An MRI magnet also irreparably damages other electrical and mechanical devices, including the following:

- Cell phones
- Pagers
- Cameras
- Calculators
- Wristwatches
- Hearing aids

Quenching. Quenching is a process by which there is a sudden loss of the superconductivity of the magnet coils so that the magnet becomes resistive. Several things may cause the magnet to quench, including the following: (1) cryogen levels get too low, (2) magnet pressure gets too high, causing higher boil-off rate of cryogens, (3) activation of the RED button on the wall inside the suite, (4) plumbing leak causing high release of cryogens or high boil-off rate, and (5) service-related problems. A controlled quench can be performed by the technologist if immediate release of the magnetic field is required due to an extreme situation such as a fire, personal safety issue, or magnet damage. Should a quench occur, helium may displace the room oxygen if it is not properly vented to the outside. Additionally, the patient and staff may suffer from suffocation and asphyxiation. This can occur very rapidly.

Safety Around Chemicals

Under OSHA guidelines, each organization is required to communicate (1) the chemical hazards in the workplace and (2) methods to protect from exposure. The Hazard Communication program is to include the following:

- Identification of hazards
- Gathering of information on the hazards
- Training of employees on correct practices
- Protective measures
- Monitoring
- Evaluation of the program

Goals of Hazard Communication Program

- To manage hazardous materials—from the point of requisition to the point of disposal—in a manner that will protect patients, visitors, and the environment from any adverse effects
- To reduce occupational illness and health problems—through education, awareness, standard operating procedures, and reduced levels of exposure (to levels as low as reasonably achievable)

Basic Components of Hazard Communication Program

Conduct an inventory of chemicals in the workplace to identify the chemical/product, location, amount, and use.

- Send the inventory electronically to the safety manager for inclusion in the organizational database
- Review labels of all chemical containers to ensure that the contents are accurately identified and provide accurate labels when necessary
- Develop a training program that includes all employees of the department and all new employees prior to their first work assignment

Training Topics in Hazard Communication Program

Employee training must include the following.

- How to obtain information about chemicals in the department inventory, or those that have been ordered or recently delivered—to include access to and use of Material Safety Data Sheets (MSDS), reference texts, and poison control center
- Hazardous properties of the chemicals inventoried—to include information on incompatible chemicals that are inventoried, what to avoid, and how to react if spills occur and chemicals mix
- Protective measures those employees must take to ensure their safety
- Emergency and immediate aid procedures if exposed—whom to contact and where to proceed if exposed or injured
- Safe handling of chemicals that are part of the employee's work responsibilities—to include a protocol review by the supervisor or lead worker
- How to clean up spills and dispose of chemicals in accordance with applicable guidelines
- Reporting to supervisor, lead worker, or Risk Management spills, exposures, or injuries
- Use of the Workers' Compensation form
- Documenting the training of all employees and the conduct of annual reviews to ensure all employees participated in the training program

Conclusion

To help maintain a safe environment for staff, patients, and visitors, your healthcare institution collaborates with several regulatory and accrediting agencies: most notably, The Joint Commission, OSHA, and CDC. As a security supervisor, you must be familiar with these outside agencies and their regulations and recommendations. The healthcare environment poses unique hazards. The stresses of coping with illness and injury can lead patients and visitors to act out in unanticipated ways. Significant exposures to blood, HIV, HBV, HCV, unrecognized tuberculosis, and other transmissible pathogens are not uncommon in this environment. The potential also exists for exposure to magnetic fields and chemicals used by ancillary departments. As a security supervisor, you must be well aware of the hazards of the environment in which you and your security staff work and the safety precautions appropriate for basic protection. To be effective and successful in healthcare security, you and your security staff must follow the basic safety protections outlined in this chapter.

Bibliography

Garner, J. S. and the Hospital Infection Control Practices Advisory Committee. Guideline for isolation precautions in hospitals. *Infect Control Hosp Epidemiol* 17(1996):53-80, and *Am J Infect Control* 24(1996):24-52. Also on the Internet, from the US Department of Health and Human Services, Centers for Disease Control and Prevention: www.cdc.gov/ncidod/dhqp/gl_isolation.html. Last modified 1 April 2005. Accessed 18 Aug 2006.

Institute for Magnetic Resonance Safety, Education, and Research (Shellock R & D Services, Inc. and F. G. Shellock). 2001. MRIsafety.com. On the Internet: www.mrisafety.com/dcfault.asp. Accessed 30 Jun 2006.

The Joint Commission. 2007. About The Joint Commission. On the Internet: www.jointcommission.org/AboutUs/. Accessed 25 May 2007.

US Department of Health and Human Services, Centers for Disease Control and Prevention. About CDC: Mission. On the Internet: www.cdc.gov/about/mission.htm. Accessed 20 Jun 2006.

US Department of Health and Human Services, Centers for Disease Control and Prevention. Standard precautions [excerpted from *Guideline for Isolation Precautions in Hospitals* (Jan 1996)]. Last modified 1 Apr 2005. On the Internet: www.cdc.gov/ncidod/dhqp/gl_isolation_standard.html. Accessed 18 Aug 2006.

US Department of Labor, Occupational Safety and Health Administration. 2006. OSHA's Mission. On the Internet: www.osha.gov/oshinfo/mission.html. Accessed 30 Jun 2006.

Study and Review Questions

1. There are several external organizations that healthcare institutions collaborate with to maintain a safe environment. What is the common mission among them?

    A. Provide training to healthcare employees

    B. Continuously promote, improve, and assure health and safety

    C. Conduct a semi-annual proactive risk assessment

    D. Regulate MRI safety

2. What is the objective of the Safety Management program?

    A. Improve organizational performance

    B. Minimize accidents and injuries

    C. Reduce or control costs for Workers' Compensation

    D. All of the above

3. Standard precautions are a set of precautions the CDC established to minimize the risk of infection. Which of the following is not covered under standard precautions?

    A. Blood and body fluids

    B. Secretions

    C. Non-intact skin

    D. Sweat

4. What is the most important concept to remember in MRI safety?

    A. The magnet is always on. It is never off. It is always a magnet.

    B. The MRI uses radio frequencies

    C. Security should never enter zone I

    D. A controlled quench can be performed by the technologist

Chapter 11

Budgeting and Cost Control

Jon Hallaway, CHPA

OBJECTIVES

After studying this chapter, the student should understand the following:

- Purpose of a budget
- Basic budget accounting terms
- General concepts of budget development
- Importance of developing and monitoring productivity standards
- Cost-reduction strategies

In the United States, the news media report almost daily that we are in a "healthcare crisis." While this "crisis" results more from problems with healthcare financing, the public is told that healthcare costs are out of control and immediate action is needed to prevent catastrophe. How long the crisis will last is unknown. But one can be assured that as long as the healthcare industry is seen to be in crisis, this issue of healthcare costs and cost control will be a major focus.

Cost control is a major concern of all healthcare executives. Healthcare organizations establish extensive budgeting programs in an attempt to anticipate costs and expected revenues. These same systems then compare actual costs incurred and revenue generated. The information is reviewed at regular intervals, often on a daily basis. Security departments are expected to provide services under the constraints of these budget guidelines.

This chapter covers the basics of healthcare security budgeting and cost control. Although you, like most supervisors, probably do not personally construct or present the budget to the administration, you need to understand the purposes of budgets and should play an integral role in budget development.

Once the budget is adopted, the job of ensuring that services are provided in the most efficient manner possible, at budgeted levels, often falls to front-line supervisors. In addition, supervisors have some of the best opportunities to improve services by bringing forth ideas to improve workplace productivity.

Since the security budget is typically presented by the security or support services management, this chapter does not discuss budget development in depth. The chapter explains basic components of the budget and how those components are developed and monitored. The supervisor's primary role—cost containment—is also addressed. Terms commonly used by finance and accounting departments appear in bold type, with a synonym or definition close by.

Budgeting

A **budget** is a financial plan. The budget projects income and expenses for a period of time. Once adopted or approved, the budget is compared against actual income and expenses at regular intervals.

A healthcare organization, like most major business operations, often has numerous departmental budgets. The departments are expected to monitor their expenses and track them against any outside income or **revenue** they might generate. Security and most of the service departments of a healthcare organization do not produce revenue (or enough revenue to offset the total costs of the department) and are classified as **cost centers**. Even if security staff is employed by a revenue-producing contract security service, the security department incurs cost; therefore, to the healthcare organization, security is a cost center.

Two Budgets: Capital and Operational

The security department typically prepares two types of budgets: capital and operational (expense) budgets.

Capital budgets are usually reserved for major purchases of equipment or systems. For capital purchases, the accounting department spreads the expense of the items over the life of the item. This **depreciation** of the item is governed by tax laws and follows a formula set by the organization. For this reason, the capital budget is kept separate from the operational budget.

Within the **operational budget,** different types of expenses are budgeted in separate **line items** or accounts. Even small security departments need to develop budgets for their salary, supply, equipment, training, and repair expense accounts. Salary expense costs are often broken down into sub-accounts (e.g., regular worked hours, overtime, and non-worked salary accounts). These accounts track the number of hours security staff is expected to work. A budget amount must be developed for each account. Those numbers must be justified and approved, and then actual performance is tracked on regular basis during the budget period.

Budget Period

The period usually covered by a budget is called the **fiscal year** (FY). The fiscal year does not necessarily start at the beginning of a calendar year. Fiscal years generally start at the beginning of a month selected by the organization and cover a 12-month period.

Budgeting Methods

Although there are several variations, most security budgets are prepared in one of two ways: traditional or **zero-based.**

The traditional method is for the organization to estimate the next year's percentage of profit or loss and then to simply increase (or decrease) each department's operating budget by that percentage. This method allows for relatively easy budget preparation and approval, but does not allow for any true growth or recognition of services.

Most organizations have moved to zero-based budgeting. In zero-based budgeting, each proposed budgeted account returns to a zero amount and all requested funds must be justified every budget year. This requires documentation to support the requested amounts for salaries, equipment, supplies, and training costs. Good documentation and presentation of the requested items for the budget often lead to success. Often, failure to do either leads to a reduced budget and lack of support from management.

Budget Development

Managers need to seek input from their supervisors to develop their budgets properly. As Harvey Burnstein notes in his book *Security, A Management Perspective,* since supervisors normally write subordinates' performance reviews, they are best positioned to know the percentage increase they will recommend. Supervisors are generally the most knowledgeable about staff training needs and, when the department must budget for tuition reimbursement, they typically know which staff members will be attending school and seeking reimbursement.

In his book *Winning,* Jack Welch comments on the budget process and how it is often dreaded by both the department and upper management. Welch observes that most budget sessions are based completely on the past year's performance. The department asks for more than it really wants and upper management tries to hold costs by trying to approve less than the department might actually need. The result is a negotiated settlement in which neither side is particularly happy.

Unfortunately, this is often the case in many institutions. A different approach to this process can benefit any department, especially the security department. As Jeff Karpovich noted in the previous edition of this manual, some administrators believe there is little or no income associated with security departments and security spending is not likely to add to the bottom line. This is a narrow view that security supervisors need to work with their manager to dispel. Karpovich's suggested approach to developing a successful security budget is outlined in the sidebar. Each aspect is discussed separately in the paragraphs that follow.

Developing a Successful Security Budget
1. Identify a need
2. Document potential expense
3. Justify the expense
4. Ensure regulatory compliance

Identify a Need

Use incident reporting, daily activity logs, hazardous surveillance feedback, and risk analysis reports to identify needs. Focus on the future plans of the department and facility. Be sure to prioritize needs and do not ask for items just because they would be nice to have.

Avoid the temptation to pad or provide a budget cushion just in case. This is not good practice for three reasons. First, funds allotted unnecessarily are not available to other departments for legitimate expenses. Second, senior management views padding as non-supportive of organization-wide objectives (the manager is not considered a team player). Third, the manager may be viewed as a poor planner.

Budget for likely needs based on current data and history. If unexpected events warrant legitimate expenses, the administration will accept unfavorable budget reports that are accompanied by documented explanations.

Document Potential Expense

Contact reputable vendors and compare prices and services. Most companies maintain a Web site with ample product information. Be sure to request quotes that will be honored when purchased in the next fiscal year or be sure to factor for inflation.

Justify the Expense

Explain why the expense is necessary and how the need was determined. Do not request an item merely because it was in last year's budget. Senior management expects and deserves a **cost-benefit analysis.** This analysis involves comparing the cost of the program or an item to its expected benefit to the organization. Do not forget that many an organization has suffered major losses from fire or water leak damages all from the want of a basic fire watch or rounds program.

Remember that the security manager must justify a capital (equipment) budget as well as an operational budget. In the healthcare organization, many departments compete for the major funds required to purchase equipment. Managers often are required to show what the return on investment **(ROI)** will be for the purchase of the item. While the return on the cost of new imaging equipment might be shown as increased revenue, the return on a major surveillance system needs to be shown differently. Security equipment purchases are usually justified by the expenses avoided, rather than revenue received. Security must be prepared to demonstrate how security expenses improve the bottom line. For example, does the expenditure help with any of the following:

- Prevent losses of the organization's property
- Control insurance premiums
- Minimize legal claims

The organization loses income *and* bears the cost of replacing the stolen item. While the savings from all these considerations may not equal the cost of a major security system, the healthcare organization must always remember the immeasurable benefit of being viewed by the public and employees as a safe place.

Ensure Regulatory Compliance

Monies requested to comply with regulatory entities and legislation contribute to budget approval. For example, expenses may be due to regulations of The Joint Commission or requirements of the Healthcare Insurance Portability and Accountability Act (HIPAA). Most administrators realize there cannot be privacy without security.

Jack Welch suggests viewing the budget process as a continual tool for monitoring and beating last year's performance. The budget should not be just a way to track costs. Rather, the budget should be part of an overall operating plan that monitors the department's performance and contribution to the overall organization's success.

Performance-based thinking might be new to many supervisors. Many may be overwhelmed with day-to-day supervision tasks (e.g., scheduling), but this outlook is critical to the success of the department. Always be aware of the need to monitor and improve workplace productivity, especially if you hope to expand services or your role in the organization.

Productivity

Productivity refers to the amount of output by an employee or business unit compared to the amount of input staffing hours needed. This output, sometimes referred to as volume, is a measure of the production or success of the employee or business unit. When a clinic increases the number of patients seen in a typical workday without increasing staffing needs, it has increased its productivity.

Measures of Productivity

To measure productivity properly, a business unit must first define the primary measures of output. The ratio of productivity is defined during the budget process and measured throughout the fiscal year. For many departments, a single item is chosen as the primary productivity measure. Additional productivity measures are often used for performance improvement initiatives or as performance incentives for managers.

The most common productivity measure for healthcare security departments (and many service departments) is square footage. For these departments, productivity is defined as follows:

$$\frac{\text{Amount of square footage protected}}{\text{Staffing hours needed to protect that area}}$$

Productivity measures are often used for performance improvement and other projects. The following are some of the more common measures of a healthcare security department's productivity:

- Security rounds conducted per shift
- Security escorts performed per day
- Security condition reports filed per officer
- Security vehicle assists per hours worked

Note that a bicycle patrol could be justified by the increases in rounds per shift of the parking areas that it provides. A security vehicle might provide that increase and more *plus* increase the number of escorts performed. Proper selection and tracking of indicators can allow you to improve and expand programs.

Process Improvement

A related concept to productivity is the **Six Sigma** philosophy of process improvement, developed by Motorola. Six Sigma seeks to eliminate defects in operations (and hence improve quality) by carefully monitoring performance data. As an example, a department could have an average response time of 3.0 minutes, yet still have some waits of 20 to 30 minutes. Those long waits would be considered defects and seen as unacceptable in a Six Sigma program.

Benchmarking

Using standard productivity measures allows your organization to benchmark against other organizations. In **benchmarking,** a best-practice standard is sought among similar healthcare standards. The best-performing facility becomes the benchmark—the standard against which the others are measured.

As healthcare organizations use more outside performance management systems, they become exposed to greater amounts of benchmarking data. This often includes a bewildering assortment of security productivity numbers from many different types of medical facilities. You and your manager need to understand what your productivity measures are being benchmarked against. An urban trauma center located in a high crime area likely requires a larger security staff than a similarly sized community hospital in a suburban setting. From a security protection standpoint, the urban hospital should not benchmark against the productivity of the community hospital.

Responsible Reporting

A supervisor able to get all assigned work done with minimum amounts of staff and overtime achieves a good productivity rating. This supervisor should be recognized for good work. A supervisor operating with low staffing levels who falsely claims that all assigned tasks were completed will also achieve a good productivity rating. But this supervisor is a risk to the organization. Not only does this unethical behavior expose the department to breach of contract or inadequate security claims, but it also creates a false impression to management that the security staff is more productive than it really is. The likely results will be difficulty justifying an increase (or even maintaining) staffing during the next budget review.

Hidden Costs
Remember that, even though your department budget may contain numerous expense accounts, major department expenses often are not shown in this budget. Benefits and the overhead costs associated with support departments, such as human resources and accounting, are often not included in the department's budget. The actual costs of a security department to the organization often go beyond the security budget. Keep in mind that you may need to justify the additional, often hidden, costs of the security department.

Monitoring
Managers usually receive financial performance data on a monthly basis. Payroll performance data may be provided on a biweekly, weekly, or even daily basis. These reports show how the department is performing compared to the original budget.

The terms "favorable to budget," "meeting budget," and being "in the black" all mean performance is good. Conversely, being "in the red" or "unfavorable" is not good, and correction will be expected.

Although supervisors need not know all budget performance data, you should receive salary, productivity, and any other budget performance information for areas under your control.

In monitoring budget data, a commonly used term is **FTE** (full-time equivalent). An FTE is determined simply by dividing the hours used in the period by a number that a single full-time employee would have worked. For example, if 168 hours were accumulated in a week, you would divide the 168 by 40 (the hours a full-time employee would work in that week) and end up with 4.2 FTEs. If only "worked hours" are calculated in the formula, the term **worked FTEs** is used. **Paid FTEs** denotes all hours recorded for the period, including holiday, sick, and vacation hours. FTE calculations are based on the actual hours budgeted or used for the period. Since this includes non-worked, part-time, and per-diem hours, understand that this number rarely equals the actual number of employees in a department.

Cost Control
Unless special approval has been given, always control costs and keep them at budgeted levels. When costs exceed budgeted guidelines, be proactive and seek to reduce expenses. Although you may be able to defer purchases of items to reduce spending, realize that salary costs are typically the main component of the security budget—generally, 80 to 85 percent and often as much as 95 percent. Supervisors soon realize that proper management of security staff provides the best means of cost control. The sidebar lists ways you can control payroll costs. Each of these is discussed in the paragraphs that follow.

> ### *Cost Control Measures Supervisors May Implement*
> - Pay close attention to overtime
> - Analyze scheduling
> - Be safe
> - Minimize turnover
> - Take proper care of equipment
> - Monitor supply costs
> - Promote security awareness
> - Consider the value-added approach

Pay Close Attention to Overtime
Overtime is one of the most expensive, and often the most visible, budget item in the security department. Whenever possible, overtime should be approved in advance and all emergency use should require approval. Doing so ensures staff do not abuse overtime.

Analyze Scheduling
You may find you do not have much flexibility with your budget, but that does not restrict you from using creative scheduling. Scheduling should be done around the needs of the organization and not based on the status quo. You can supplement traditional 8-hour shifts with 10-hour or 12-hour swing shifts to create "compressed" schedules and allow for additional staffing at key overlap times.

Often, you can increase employee morale with creative scheduling since some staff members may prefer a four-day work week.

Be Safe
The cost of benefits for employees injured on the job may not be shown on the department budget, but is a major expense to the organization. Encourage safe work practices in all aspects of the job.

Minimize Turnover
Turnover costs money. Recruitment, using overtime to cover vacancies, and training are all expenses that might be avoided. Effective use of supervision and management techniques covered in this manual benefit both the supervisor and the organization in hiring and retaining quality staff members. Retention of quality staff allows for a high level of service and saves money.

Take Proper Care of Equipment
Costs of repair and replacement of patrol vehicles, golf carts, and alarm monitoring equipment can be deferred if staff members take proper care of department equipment. Always be alert for indications of negligence or abuse.

Monitor Supply Costs
Even though supply expenses might be a comparatively small portion of the security budget, supplies must be properly used and managed. Any impression of misappropriation, waste, or misuse appears negatively to the administration and may cause problems with budget reviews.

Do not forget the need for all staff members to be alert to the cost savings of turning off lights and appliances not in use, identifying over- and under-heated or air-conditioned spaces, and preventing unnecessary vehicle idling. While these may not directly benefit the bottom line of the security department, promoting these types of actions earns the security department a reputation as an attention-to-detail team player.

Promote Security Awareness
Getting others involved creates a safer environment and allows for a more productive security force. An alert and aware staff of employees and volunteers deters many incidents and creates apprehension in others.

Consider the Value-added Approach
In value-added programs, security takes on expanded roles in non-traditional security responsibilities. These might include greater responsibilities with life safety, PBX operations (phones), patient escorts, maintenance, and staff transportation. You are wise to use surplus time or surplus staffing for value-added programs.

Strategies for Contract Supervisors
Contract supervisors sometimes find themselves in a difficult situation as they work to control costs for the client while recommending increased service expenditures that would increase the contract company's revenues. By practicing the cost control suggestions outlined in this section, contract supervisors and staff gain the trust of facility administration. As a result, appropriation requests, including additional contract officers, are not viewed as self-serving and are a crucial step to building a successful contract relationship.

Cost-Reduction Strategies

Sometimes, economic conditions require reductions greater than can be achieved by simple cost controls. When major reductions in security expenses are needed, the strategies listed in the sidebar must be considered. Each of these is discussed separately in the paragraphs that follow.

> ### Cost-reduction Strategies
> ### When Major Reductions Are Needed
> - Re-classify posts or positions
> - Outsource
> - Balance labor with technology
> - Downsize

Re-classification of Posts or Positions
Certain posts may suffice with a less trained, lower paid employee. Hiring a parking attendant instead of a highly trained security officer to serve as a gate guard may be a better use of resources. Temporary employees for some areas may also be a cost-effective option.

Outsourcing
Using contract staff to supplement in-house forces has worked well for many facilities. These hybrid programs work especially well when the program calls for fluctuating staffing levels due to construction or other programs.

Balancing Labor with Technology
Proper use of technology can replace staffing in some instances. This must be approached carefully, since adding non-integrated security controls often results in an opposite need to add staff. Do not ever believe the technology can replace staffing completely. Someone needs to monitor equipment, and staff must respond to and verify breaches or alarm conditions. Most municipalities have ordinances restricting organizations from pushing these responsibilities completely on local law enforcement.

Reduction in Force
A harsh reality, layoffs (or a reduction in force) are a part of business. Communicate with your managers to retain the most qualified officers. Also ask if **attrition,** the act of not replacing a voluntarily vacated position, is an option in place of a reduction in force.

Conclusion
The rise in healthcare consumerism has driven many healthcare organizations to seek better ways to improve service and convenience and control costs (Frampton 2003). Service departments, traditionally viewed as "fixed" in expenditures and service, are now being asked to align their services and strategies to that of the healthcare organization as a whole. Security departments must design and budget their programs around the goals of the organization and then monitor that performance on a regular basis. With a primary view to protecting the assets of the facility, the security department must be prepared to take on a greater and more productive role in helping the organization meet its goals.

Bibliography
Burnstein, H. 1996. *Security, A Management Perspective.* Englewood Cliffs, NJ: Prentice Hall.

Frampton, S., L. Gilpin and P. A. Charmel. 2003. *Putting Patients First.* San Francisco: Jossey Bass.

Welch, J. 2005. *Winning.* New York: Harper Collins.

Study and Review Questions

1. What is a budget?
   - A. Financial plan
   - B. Expense projection
   - C. Revenue projection
   - D. List of cost centers

2. Define ROI.
   - A. Return on income
   - B. Return on investment
   - C. Revenue on investment
   - D. Revenue on income

3. What does benchmarking accomplish?
   - A. Evaluates performance
   - B. Estimates productivity
   - C. Establishes a best-practice standard
   - D. Reviews square footage and productivity

4. Which of the following is not a cost control measure?
   - A. Analyze scheduling
   - B. Pay close attention to overtime
   - C. Monitor supply costs
   - D. Increase expenses

5. What is the act of not replacing a voluntarily vacated position called?
   - A. Reduction in force
   - B. Attrition
   - C. Layoffs
   - D. Reclassifying positions

Chapter 12

Principles of Customer Service

Robert "Mickey" Watson, CHPA

OBJECTIVES

After studying this chapter, the student should understand the following:

- The broad definition of the term "customer" as it relates to the security officer and the security management program
- How to build a culture of outstanding customer service within the security program
- How customer interactions with the security department impact the organization as a whole
- How to evaluate the department, subordinates, and one's self for customer relations effectiveness

The terms "security" and "customer relations" are not often used in the same sentence. Many in the healthcare setting think of security as the department that deals only with problems, crime, and disruptive patients and visitors. Security is often thought of as the tool to use when customer relations have failed. Nothing could be further from the truth. The security department is in many cases, the organization's front line in the realm of customer relations. The security officer is often the first individual with whom a customer comes into contact and, in many cases, the last person the customer sees when departing the facility. Simply seeing a neat, uniformed, and approachable security officer at an entrance can be a huge step in providing effective customer service. When the customer feels safe, the entire customer experience is affected in a positive way. As a security supervisor, your role is to empower and instruct the security officers in your department on the appropriate customer service standards and methods used at your organization.

Recognize Your Customers

To cultivate effective customer relations and provide outstanding customer service, you must first be able to define the term "customer."

Customers come in many shapes, sizes, colors, and origins. Patients are definitely customers, as are patients' family members and visitors. But what about the board member, chief executive officer, staff member, contractor, volunteer, homeless man, or alcoholic who shows up nightly in the emergency department? They are all customers, too. Customers are every single human being with whom we come into contact in the course of our duties.

External and Internal Customers

Customers can be divided into two distinct categories. Recognize that you have both external and internal customers.

- ***External Customers:*** Patients, visitors, family members, vendors, law enforcement, and other public safety professionals are some of your external customers. Anyone with whom you or other staff members have contact who is not a member of, or affiliated with, the organization is considered an external customer.

- **Internal Customers:** Physicians, administrators, board members, volunteers, contractors, and all other staff members are your internal customers.

A Supportive Culture

Customer service in its simplest terms mirrors the Golden Rule: Do unto others as you would have them do unto you. Treat each person as you would want to be treated. Ask yourself, "If this were my mother, how would I respond to her needs?"

Healthcare organizations that rate among the best in the nation cultivate a culture of customer service throughout their organization. Each and every member of the team recognizes the importance of their contribution to the overall customer service experience. They themselves are customers of the organization and of every other member of the team. Great customer relations start at the very top of the organization and cascade down like a waterfall. Every person in the chain passes it on.

Customer Service Fundamentals

Many times, parents, grandparents, and older co-workers talk about "the good old days." They speak of a time when people put others first, took the time to help a neighbor, and were concerned about being polite. Today's fast pace is a result of technology, the pursuit of profit, and the never-ending drive to do it faster. To return to the basics, you and your staff must re-examine the rules of customer service. Strong customer service is a business essential. Providing this service is not as difficult if you and your employees follow some basic rules on customer service. The Web site AllBusiness.com lists and describes these basic rules of customer service:

- Commit to quality service
- Know your products
- Know your customers
- Treat people with courtesy and respect
- Never argue with a customer

- Do not leave customers in limbo
- Always provide what you promise
- Assume that your customers tell the truth
- Focus on making customers—not on sales
- Make it easy to buy

Although targeted to sales, these rules easily apply to the practice of healthcare security. Consider how each can and should be implemented and emphasized by staff in your organization.

Customer Relations Impact

First impressions set the tone for the entire visit. Imagine pulling up to the curb of a hospital emergency department at 2:30 a.m. Your loved one in the vehicle is very ill. The first person you see is a healthcare security officer. The officer's actions at this moment may very well define your entire experience with the facility. Did the officer offer assistance or look the other way? Was the officer polite and caring or rude and indifferent? Was the officer neat and clean or in a rumpled, ill-fitting uniform? The answers to these types of questions are critical in evaluating the impact of customer service initiatives within your department. The feedback received from customers should be evaluated and used to improve the service provided to everyone.

Strategies for Supervisors

The suggestions noted in the sidebar may help you improve the customer service image of your department. You must work with your officers and provide them with the necessary skills to be able to deliver good service.

Chapter 12: Principles of Customer Service

> *Emphasizing Customer Service: Strategies for Supervisors*
>
> - *Lead by Example:* Subordinates tend to treat others the way they see their supervisor treat those around them. They are also influenced by the way they are treated by their supervisor.
>
> - *Keep Up Appearances:* Nothing tarnishes the image of a security department faster than a sloppy, disheveled officer and uniform. Remember the maxim, "You only have one chance to make a first impression." Inspect your officers regularly. Develop a departmental dress code and grooming standard, and stick to it.
>
> - *Set the Bar High:* Do more than just the minimum required. Set an expectation of outstanding customer service. Hold your subordinates and yourself accountable to that standard.
>
> - *Stay Involved:* Involve yourself and the department in customer service projects and initiatives of the organization. Be on the front lines when it comes to customer service. Those whom you lead will soon follow.
>
> - *Keep Customer Service in Sight:* Make sure that discussions of successes and opportunities in customer relations are a regular topic in your meetings with staff. This cannot be a once-a-year review. Customer relations have to become the way you conduct business.
>
> - *Create the Culture:* Realize that creating a culture of outstanding customer relations is a long-term commitment. This cultural change does not happen overnight. You must celebrate your victories one at a time. Share your successes with the officers and others. Human nature seeks public praise.

Evaluating Your Customer Relations Quotient

To realize your personal potential for outstanding customer relations and customer service, start with a critical self analysis. When you want to see how your hair or uniform looks, you look in the mirror. You might also ask others, "how does my hair look today?" Similarly, you cannot determine how you are doing in your profession or other areas of life without exploring them from internal and external perspectives.

"Without getting constant feedback and input from those you are serving, you will never get better and never be able to compete in any type of marketplace. Self-evaluation is all about learning, growing, and getting better," notes Pamela Beitlich, RN, MSN, and nationally recognized customer service consultant for The Studer Group (in a conversation with this chapter's author). "But even more important than this," continues Beitlich, "in the healthcare industry, without critical self-evaluation, you will lose a wonderful opportunity to make a difference in someone's life, when they need it most."

As a security supervisor, you need to assess not only how well you are able to meet customer needs, but also how well your staff meets customer needs. The sidebar lists four tools your department can use to evaluate its customer relations. Each tool is discussed separately in the paragraphs that follow.

> *Tools to Evaluate Customer Relations*
> - Internal satisfaction surveys
> - Patient satisfaction surveys
> - Polling other leaders in the organization
> - Conducting "one on ones" with security staff

Internal Satisfaction Surveys

If your organization does not conduct overall internal satisfaction surveys, consider designing your own. Keep it simple and straightforward. Your information technology department may be able to help you create a Web- or Intranet-based survey.

Patient Satisfaction Surveys

If at all possible, include a question related to security in the patient satisfaction survey. Stay informed as to when these surveys are being updated. This is the time to make your case for inclusion in the survey.

Polling Organizational Leaders

You can conduct polls both formally and informally. Conducting a formal telephone or e-mail survey of the organizational leadership is one example. Simply asking for constructive opinion in casual conversation is an effective informal way of gathering information.

"One on Ones" with Security Staff

One-on-one conversation is the most effective tool for assessing internal satisfaction with subordinate and supervisory staff. Regular, effective, and confidential communication with staff provides a clear picture of internal satisfaction within the work group. Do not wait until problems arise to conduct this kind of self-examination. Be proactive in providing opportunities for staff to voice their opinions, successes, and concerns.

Conclusion

While our primary focus as healthcare security professionals is to *protect*, we must begin by learning to *serve*. Service builds trust, which strengthens customer confidence in our ability to protect. Security is the front line for the healthcare organization in many ways, and chief among them is customer service.

As a supervisor, you improve your department's customer service skills by ongoing management and interaction. You must provide continuous support and guidance on how to conduct effective customer service and what it means. Keep a finger on the pulse of how your officers are interacting with customers and help strengthen your program as appropriate.

For More Information

Morris, R. J. 2007. "Customer relations: public, employee, and labor relations." In *Basic Training Manual for Healthcare Security Officers*. Meserve, E. (ed.). Glendale Heights, Ill: International Association for Healthcare Security and Safety.

References

Ten rules for customer service. On the Internet: www.allbusiness.com/sales/customer-service/1023-1.html. Accessed 6 Jul 2007.

Study and Review Questions

1. What are the two categories of customers?

    A. Internal and external

    B. Internal and visitors

    C. External and physicians

    D. Vendors and patients

2. Which best defines good customer service?

    A. Customer service only needs to be done at the top of the organization

    B. Treat each person as you want to be treated

    C. Treat each person differently

    D. Customer service starts with the line employee

3. Which type of conversation is the most beneficial in assessing how you are doing with customer relations?

    A. Group

    B. One on one

    C. Team

    D. None of the above

4. Which of the following is not a recommended method of improving the customer service image of your department?

    A. Lead by example

    B. Set the bar high

    C Stay involved

    D. Sloppy appearance

Chapter 13

Professionalism and Ethics

John Driscoll, CHPA, CPP

Objectives

After studying this chapter, the student should understand the following:

- What constitutes a profession
- The importance of professional development in healthcare security
- The role the IAHSS and International Healthcare Security and Safety Foundation have taken in establishing professional status for healthcare protection services
- The need for uniform standards and regulation in the security field
- The importance of continuing education in career development
- What needs to be done for healthcare security to attain professional status

Webster's *New Collegiate Dictionary* defines professionalism as "the conduct, aims, or qualities that characterize or mark a profession or a professional person" and as "the following of a profession...for gain or livelihood." Some universally recognized professions are law, medicine, nursing, and teaching, but what constitutes a profession? The Wikipedia Web site defines a profession as "an occupation that requires extensive training and the study and mastery of specialized knowledge, and usually has a professional association, ethical code, and process of certification or licensing." In *Hospital and Healthcare Security and Safety* (Colling 2001, p. 54), Russell Colling, founding president of the IAHSS, summarizes the generally accepted criteria of a profession (see sidebar). The words "profession" and "professional" come from the Latin word *professio*, which means a public declaration with the force of promise. Colling states that the term "professional security officer" is frequently used to denote superior effort rather than to define a true professional (Colling 2001, p. 53).

Characteristics of the Professions

- Have a basis of systemic defined theory
- Have an authority recognized by those being served
- Have broad community sanction and approval of this authority
- Have a code of ethics
- Have a professional culture sustained by formal professional associations

Source: Colling, R. L. 2001. *Hospital and Healthcare Security and Safety*, 4th ed. Boston: Butterworth-Heinemann, p. 54.

Reaching Professional Status

Louis Tyska and Lawrence Fennelly, in *150 Things You Should Know About Security*, hold that these are two of the biggest obstacles to acceptance of security as a profession:

- Erroneous perceptions of the field
- Lack of a structured prerequisite to practice

Both of these obstacles are especially relevant to healthcare security. Erroneous perceptions of the security function abound throughout healthcare. In most states, no prerequisites to practice exist other than being employed by a healthcare facility or a contract security services provider.

Role of the IAHSS

The American Society for Industrial Security (now ASIS International) was organized in 1955 to establish security as a recognized profession in both government and private industry. Since then, many other security organizations have been founded to serve the specialized needs of various industries. One, the International Association for Hospital Security (now IAHSS), was chartered in 1968 and has now grown to 1688 members internationally. Via the IAHSS's chapters, members can regularly meet and exchange ideas. The association also holds seminars and hosts an annual general meeting each June. Over the years, the IAHSS has established a professional culture sustained by formal professional associations—this is one of the criteria for security to be defined as a profession.

Certifications

To ensure that each role within the healthcare security field has demonstrated skill competencies, the IAHSS has developed training certifications. The concept of professional certification is widely accepted in the healthcare industry, with certification programs in virtually every medical and ancillary field. Numerous studies have shown that professional certification is rewarded by increased compensation and more rapid advancement.

In the mid-1970s, the IAHSS first adopted a Basic Training program for hospital security officers. This training program eventually became a certification program in which applicants were required to pass an examination. The Supervisory Training program followed and then the Safety (now Health and Safety) training program and the Advanced Officer training program in 2000.

"IAHSS Certified" insignia are available to those who successfully complete each training program. The insignia are worn on the uniforms of many healthcare security and safety officers as evidence of their professional training.

In 1982, the IAHSS established the International Healthcare Security and Safety Foundation (IHSSF) to function as an education and credentialing entity for IAHSS members. The IHSSF established the professional designation of Certified Healthcare Protection Administrator (CHPA). The CHPA has been transferred to the IAHSS. There are now two steps in the CHPA credentialing program: the Graduate level and the Fellowship level.

Graduate Level. Applicants are required to have obtained qualifying credits based on their education, specialized training, and experience and to pass a written examination on four areas of expertise: management, emergency preparedness (which recently replaced risk management), security, and safety. Successful completion of this examination results in the awarding of the CHPA designation. CHPAs must be recertified every three years based on continuing education, training, and professional activities.

Fellowship Level. To earn this designation, CHPAs are required to complete a research project and write a dissertation on a healthcare security or safety subject. Applicants must then defend their paper before a committee of the board. Accepted dissertations are published by the IHASS and become part of the profession's systemic knowledge—in this way, the security profession meets another mark of a profession.

Systemic Knowledge

With the publication of the *Journal of Healthcare Protection Management* in 1984, the IAHSS began compiling the profession's systemic knowledge in a biannual journal. Articles published in the journal are indexed. Specific topics can be researched via the journal index on the IAHSS Web site. Another component of this systemic knowledge is the bank of healthcare security policies and procedures and basic industry guidelines available from IAHSS headquarters.

Ethics

Ethical conduct is a prerequisite for any person who aspires to professional status; however, ethical conduct is even more important in the security/protection field due to the trust placed in a security officer by the employing institution.

The *Encyclopedia of Security Management* states that "The security manager encounters ethics in two dimensions: first, as the employer's instrument for developing business conduct policy and investigating improper conduct by others; and second, as an employee who is personally obligated to conduct business in accordance with the established policy" (Fay 1993).

Some of the unethical actions a supervisor needs to be aware of include kickbacks, distributing proprietary information, and conflicts of interest. Supervisors must be aware of possible unethical behaviors and know how to deal with an issue once identified. Healthcare security executives must ensure that their institutions have specific policy guidance, monitoring, and enforcement in these and other areas of ethical concern.

In 1981, the IAHSS first adopted a Code of Ethics applicable to its members. Since then, only minor changes have been made in what has become the ethical standard for past, present, and future healthcare security administrators (see sidebar).

INTERNATIONAL ASSOCIATION FOR HEALTHCARE SECURITY AND SAFETY

Code of Ethics

Preamble: "Recognizing that the overall quality of healthcare delivery is directly related to the professional services rendered by the International Association for Healthcare Security and Safety, the following Code of Ethics is hereby mandated as a consideration for membership."

As a healthcare security professional, I pledge to dedicate myself to providing a safe and secure environment to the people and institution(s) I serve by:

- Supporting patient care and awareness within my healthcare facility
- Recognizing that my principal responsibilities are security and safety services to the healthcare community that I serve
    - to protect life and property and reduce crime through the implementation of recognized crime prevention and investigative techniques, and
    - to provide a safe environment of care in support of the mission of the healthcare facility
- Respecting the moral and constitutional rights of all persons while performing my duties without prejudice
- Ensuring that confidential and privileged information is protected at all times
- Maintaining open communication with other professionals with whom I conduct business
- Striving to further my education, both academically and technically, while encouraging professional development and/or advancement of other security/safety personnel
- Promoting and exemplifying the highest standards of integrity to those whom I serve while dedicating myself to my chosen profession

The IAHSS Code of Ethics fulfills another criteria required of a profession—that of a code of ethics.

Regulation

An obstacle to recognition of security as a practice, note Tyska and Fennelly, is the lack of a structured prerequisite to practice. Most recognized professionals (e.g., accountants, attorneys, nurses, physicians, psychologists, teachers) are regulated by either state governments or, in some cases (e.g., attorneys), professional associations. As a prerequisite for licensure, regulations for professions typically always require the first two items listed below and usually also require the third:

- Complete a specified academic or vocational training program as a prerequisite for licensure
- Adhere to a code of ethics
- Pass a written examination

The regulatory or licensing authority may revoke a license to practice for violation of state law, its regulations, or its code of ethics.

Since the 1960s, most states license or certify public safety workers (e.g., police officers, firefighters, emergency medical technicians). However, few states license security officers unless they are armed and/or employees of contract security companies. In most states, contract security companies are licensed, but proprietary security organizations (e.g., healthcare security departments consisting entirely of in-house employees) are not regulated.

Published Recommendations

Government and public awareness of this lack of regulation began in 1971 with the publication of the RAND report on *Private Police in the United States*, vol. I. This report led to formation of the Task Force on Security of the National Advisory Committee on Criminal Justice Standards and Goals, funded by the Law Enforcement Assistance Administration of the US Department of Justice. In 1976, the task force released the 580-page *Report of the Task Force on Private Security*. This report recommended significant changes in the hiring, training, and employment of security officers and included model legislation. The vast majority of these recommendations were not adopted.

Additional efforts aimed at setting standards for private security have included the following:

- The 1985 *Hallcrest Report* specifically acknowledged "the certification efforts of the International Association for Hospital Security (which) have made a significant contribution to the training of security personnel working in healthcare facilities."
- In April 2002, the Private Liaison Committee of the International Association of Chiefs of Police proposed standards for private security officers (IACP 2002).
- In 2003, ASIS International's Commission on Guidelines released draft selection and training guidelines for private security officers. Significantly, these guidelines do not go far beyond those recommended by the *Report of the Task Force on Private Security* nearly 30 years ago.

Most security professionals in healthcare recognize and support the need for uniform standards and regulation in the security field. While the IAHSS has been in the forefront of efforts to train and certify healthcare security officers and credential healthcare security executives, these programs will not become universally accepted unless required by state laws and regulations.

Education

Academic Programs

Most recognized professions require specific academic training—at least an undergraduate (bachelor's) degree. Although healthcare security has no such requirements, an increasing number of healthcare facilities require an undergraduate or in some cases a graduate (master's) degree to be eligible for security management positions. Associate degrees in security and loss prevention are offered by many community colleges, and a number of colleges and universities offer a bachelor's degree in security administration or in criminal justice with a concentration in security administration.

In the 1990s, ASIS International embarked on a partnership with Webster University to offer a graduate degree in security administration at locations throughout the United States. With the dramatic expansion of distance learning on the Internet, both undergraduate and graduate degree programs in security are accessible to healthcare security professionals virtually anywhere in the world.

When considering a distance education program, you must first differentiate between accredited and unaccredited programs. As well, steer clear of "diploma mills" that advertise credit for life experience and degrees up to and including a PhD without completing any classes. Such degrees not only do not expand your professional horizons, but also are a sure way to have your résumé disregarded by knowledgeable human resources recruiters.

Most healthcare facilities encourage employees at all levels to continue their education. Many offer tuition assistance or reimbursement for courses taken from accredited institutions. The healthcare security professional not only takes advantage of these opportunities, but also encourages subordinates to do so. The importance of education to healthcare security professionals can best be illustrated by recognizing that over 60 percent of the personnel in most healthcare organizations (physicians and nurses) are degreed professionals. They worked hard for their degrees and will respect those in other professions who have taken the time and effort to do likewise.

Industry Programs

In addition to academic degrees, numerous educational programs are offered by professional associations in both security and healthcare. For example:

- *Security Industry:* ASIS International's many educational offerings give security personnel in all fields the knowledge and tools they need to function effectively in a corporate environment.
- *Healthcare Industry:* In healthcare, organizations such as the American College of Healthcare Executives (ACHE) offer courses in various aspects of healthcare administration. These enable security managers to think globally instead of just in terms of security.

Taking advantage of these educational opportunities prepares security personnel for advancement into senior management positions with increased responsibilities.

Contributions to Professionalism

Theodore Roosevelt once said that, "Every man owes something to the advancement of his profession." As security professionals, we owe a great deal to our profession, and each of us has an obligation to advance it by developing our subordinates as well as ourselves. We must be active in professional associations such as the IAHSS, share our experiences by writing for publications such as the *Journal of Healthcare Protection Management,* and work to enact meaningful legislation to provide for the effective regulation of the security profession. Only when healthcare security has achieved full recognition as a profession will we achieve status and compensation compatible with our responsibilities.

References

Colling, R. L. 2001. *Hospital and Healthcare Security*, 4th ed. Boston: Butterworth-Heinemann, pp. 53–54.

Cunningham, W. C., T. H. Taylor and Hallcrest Systems, Inc. 1985. *The Hallcrest Report: Private Security and Police in America*. Portland, Ore: Chancellor Press.

Fay, J. J. 1993. *Encyclopedia of Security Management*. Boston: Butterworth-Heinemann, p. 97.

Kakalik, J. S. and S. Wildhorn. 1971. *Private Police in the United States*, vol. 1 *(Rand report)*. Santa Monica: Rand Corp.

Merriam-Webster's Collegiate Dictionary, 11th ed. 2003. Springfield, Mass: Merriam-Webster, Inc.

Private Security Liaison Committee. 2002. Private security officer selection, training, licensing guidelines. Alexandria, Va: International Association of Chiefs of Police. On the Internet: www.theiacp.org/documents/pdfs/Publications/privatesecurityofficer&2Epdf. Accessed 19 Jun 2007.

Task Force on Security of the National Advisory Committee on Criminal Justice Standards and Goals. 1976. Report of the Task Force on Private Security. Washington, DC: Law Enforcement Assistance Administration, US Department of Justice.

Tyska, L. A. and L. J. Fennelly. 1998. *150 Things You Should Know About Security*. Boston: Butterworth-Heineman, p. 157.

Wikipedia. Last modified 30 May 2007. Profession (Web page). On the Internet: http:/en.wikipedia.org/wiki/Profession. Accessed 19 Jun 2007.

Bibliography

Cassidy-Ervin, D. Feb 1989. Ethically speaking… *Security Management*, pp. 99–100.

Davies, S. J. and R. R. Minion. 1995. *The Security Supervisor Training Manual*. Boston: Butterworth-Heinemann.

Fay, J. J. 1993. *Encyclopedia of Security Management*. Boston: Butterworth-Heinemann, p. 97.

Hill, I. July 1981. Common sense and everyday ethics. *Security Management*, pp. 123–132.

Wanat, J., E. Guy and J. Merrigan. 1981. *Supervisory Techniques for the Security Professional*. Boston: Butterworth.

Chapter 13: Professionalism and Ethics

Study and Review Questions

1. Which of the following defines professionalism?

    A. The conduct or qualities that characterize or mark a profession

    B. A basis of systemic theory

    C. A code of ethics

    D. Superior effort

2. What are the two biggest obstacles to security being accepted as a profession?

    A. No code of ethics and lack of a structured prerequisite to practice

    B. Lack of a structured prerequisite to practice and erroneous perceptions of the field

    C. Erroneous perceptions of the field and no code of ethics

    D. Lack of superior effort and lack of structured prerequisite to practice

3. How many levels exist in the CHPA credentialing program?

    A. Three

    B. One

    C. Two

    D. Four

4. Which training program was developed by the IAHSS first?

    A. Supervisor

    B. Advanced

    C. Health and safety

    D. Basic

Chapter 14

Effective Crime Prevention Programs

Bryan Warren, CHPA

OBJECTIVES

After studying this chapter, the student should understand the following:

- How crime prevention programs can enhance an existing security department
- How to create and implement crime prevention programs
- The importance of these programs in preventing security-related incidents

---

Crime prevention programs are one of the most useful value-added services your department can offer. These programs are also one of the easiest value-added services to implement. Crime prevention programs enhance the security department's value to the organization. They also educate scores of employees in proper methods to reduce crime and security-related incidents. Involving facility employees in crime prevention extends the eyes and ears of the security team.

As a supervisor in security, you have the opportunity and responsibility to identify suitable topics for crime prevention programs that can help your organization. You must determine what types of programs to offer, in what format, when. You must locate and apply resources. The task entails weighing the advantages and disadvantages of using internal staff, external providers, or a combination thereof. Tapping into the knowledge and resources of other departments is advised. So, too, is drawing from professional associations, publications, and government resources. An array of useful information is available, often for free. Most of all, your crime prevention programs must be of interest and help to those your department serves.

Identifying Program Topics

Employee surveys and security incident reports are two tools useful for identifying topics of concern in your facility. Awareness of recurring, seasonal problems can help you schedule timely programs that help deter crime. One topic that is applicable to all employees is how and when to contact security.

Conducting Surveys

One way to get a feel for what might work best in your environment is to conduct a brief employee survey and review the results. Have security personnel survey employees in various departments and on all shifts about their concerns regarding security-related matters. Ask what educational offerings are of interest.

The answers might surprise you. Many security professionals think healthcare employees are mostly worried about workplace violence and the like. The survey might show you that issues such as identity theft or petty theft are also of concern.

Analyzing Incident Reports

Incident reports can reveal important topics for crime prevention programs. Review your security incident reports for trends or patterns. You may note a high number of thefts from one department or a parking lot, or you may find an increase in the number of thefts of laptop computers. Use the results to determine what will make the most impact.

Addressing Seasonal Concerns

Certain topics are somewhat seasonal. The fall and winter months are a good time to discuss personal safety tips. (Daylight savings time is over so the days get darker sooner; also many people are doing holiday shopping so theft of goods and money is more of a concern.) Spring and summer are ripe for discussions of de-escalation. (Hotter temperatures often mean hotter heads.)

Identifying Resources

In-house or Out-sourced?

You can use internal or external resources to develop and offer the crime prevention programs you need. The decision on whether to out-source or use in-house staff can depend on several factors. The most obvious consideration is what type of security force your organization has.

If the security force is proprietary, examine the pros and cons of using an in-house staff member and researcher to develop and offer a specific program. If a contract agency provides your security force, ask if they offer such programs or might be willing to have an employee assist in creating and presenting a program. A third alternative is to hire an outside consultant to create a program that fits your needs. The table lists some advantages and disadvantages of in-house versus out-sourced programs.

Advantages & Disadvantages: In-house vs. Out-sourced Programs

In-house
Advantages:
• Program may cost less
• Staff member may be known, or become known, to many employees
Disadvantages:
• Requires an investment in time: staff must develop and present material

Out-sourced
Advantages:
• Program is already developed; little or no research is required
Disadvantages:
• Program may be costly
• You may not have as much control over content

Important: Only you can determine if the knowledge, skills, and resources of an out-sourced presenter and program developer would exceed those of in-house staff and more effectively accomplish your goals.

Ensuring Valuable Content

Especially if you decide to use an outside consultant or agency to create a program, address the following up front to ensure the program will be of value:

- *Appropriate Intensity:* An over-enthusiastic presenter may frighten people by telling vivid stories of assaults or worse. Usually, this occurs just before the instructor offers a deal on pepper spray or personal alarms.
- *Healthcare Focus:* Programs designed for another type of business might not translate easily into material appropriate for healthcare security. Find out what employees in your organization are looking for in a security-related educational offering.
- *Referrals:* Ask for references from candidates who wish to provide such classes. Contact their previous clients for feedback. A good question to ask is, "Would you consider having them back to teach at your organization again?" If the answer is no, continue your search.

Creating Your Own Program

Creating a crime prevention program is not the daunting task that it might seem.

- Look at the results of your initial data gathering (e.g., survey, incident reports) to see what people want to know more about
- Choose a topic that most can relate to and appreciate, such as personal safety tips
- Research this topic

Tapping Available Resources

Be sure to use professional resources to help develop the program's content. Tap the resources within your healthcare organization and external resources within security and related professions. Look also for information from government agencies.

External Resources. Use professional publications, the Internet, local law enforcement agencies, and peers in the healthcare security community, such as your local chapter of the IAHSS.

Internal Resources. For specialized programs, such as workplace violence prevention, get assistance from departments in your organization that deal with the issue. Two examples are given here:

- The human resources department can discuss the zero tolerance workplace violence policy that most organizations have
- The employee assistance program can discuss what types of counseling and assistance can be provided to victims of workplace violence

Multi-disciplinary Approach. The crime prevention programs you offer should be pertinent to any security-related issues that may be occurring at your organization. As you design these programs, be sure to tap into the resources within your organization. Enlist other employees and departments in information gathering and developing the educational program. See the sidebar for an example. By taking a multi-disciplinary approach, you share the research and course preparation workload while involving other departments in security-related training.

In Developing Programs, Take a Multi-disciplinary Approach

Example: Preventing Theft of Laptop Computers

Your organization may have had a lot of laptop computers stolen lately. To put together an educational program to address issues related to this problem, you could do the following:

1. Contact the Information Services/ Information Technology department (IS/IT).

    Get input on why certain computers make better targets that others (such as laptops are more portable and easier to resell). Solicit advice on how to prevent such thefts (most organizations have policies in place regarding specific standards for securing such equipment).

2. Talk to the coordinator for risk management and standards relevant to the Health Insurance Portability and Accountability Act (HIPAA).

    Discuss the loss of not only the computer, but of the information that it might contain (possibly leading to identity theft or litigation against the organization).

3. Look at your recent incidents of laptop theft.

    Note how these thefts occurred (e.g., offices left unattended and unsecured, laptops left in personal vehicles in plain sight).

Explaining these three facets gives you at least a one-hour program on how to prevent future laptop thefts. The program will use not only your expertise in physical security, but also the knowledge of the IS/IT and risk management departments. Risk management staff may even assist by getting this information into a PowerPoint for you. And IS/IT may be able to advertise the program on the organization's Intranet.

Each of your departments has its own specialty, so why not use them all for a common goal?

Choosing an Appropriate Format

Consider the format of the program. Some ideas are given below. What would best suit the intended audience and the topic you wish to cover? Will employees have questions, or do you need merely to give them information.

- *Formal Lecture:* A speaker can address a large audience. A PowerPoint presentation can be an affective aid. A presentation developed in-house may later be viewed online or made available on video.
- *Small, Informal Gathering:* A focused program can be provided to an individual department or section of the organization. A "lunch and learn" program is one example.
- *Self-paced Learning:* Crime prevention information can be easily disseminated to the entire staff at once. Employees can then review the information at their convenience. Vehicles for self-paced learning include self-learning modules and newsletters.
- *Online Information:* Information offered online (through the organization's computer network) might include organization policies and procedures, announcements, and information about new services. This is a great vehicle for crime prevention programs.
- *Traditional Communication Vehicles:* Bulletin boards and flyers work well for disseminating information, especially at facilities with a smaller workforce. Newsletters and payroll "stuffers" also are effective.

Offering Problem-oriented Programs

If there is a specific topic that requires additional staff education or a certain issue that needs addressing, a problem-oriented program may be in order. For example, you may have an increase in the theft of unattended purses or a rash of laptop computer thefts. A problem-oriented program can address the issue. Some examples are given below.

Theft from Autos

You can deter thefts from autos by educating employees not to leave valuables in plain sight inside their vehicles. Create colorful "Make Your Vehicle A Hard Target" citations. Security can complete the citations and leave them on the windshields of employee vehicles.

Unattended Items

Similarly, you can issue notices whenever unattended and unsecured areas or items are discovered by security patrols. This not only educates the employees not to repeat this behavior, but also indicates that security has been patrolling the area in question.

Multi-disciplinary Taskforce

You can create a multi-disciplinary taskforce to address specific issues, such as workplace violence or theft prevention.

Plainclothes Security Surveillance

You can set up surveillance in selected areas, for example in an area where there have been repeated thefts.

Conclusion

Security in a healthcare environment is every employee's responsibility. By teaming up with other departments and offering proactive ways to reduce unwanted incidents, your security department can easily provide value-added service to the organization. Keep your eyes and ears open for crime prevention programs appropriate to create and offer for your organization. Doing so helps everyone deter crime.

Bibliography

Fennelly, L. J. 1999. *Handbook of Loss Prevention and Crime Prevention*, 3rd ed. Boston: Butterworth-Heinemann.

Gray, R. 2006 Nov/Dec. Extreme makeover: hospital edition. *Campus Safety*. On the Internet: www.campussafetymagazine.com/Articles/?ArticleID=71. Accessed 13 Mar 2007.

Sennewald, C. A. 1998. *Effective Security Management*, 3rd ed. Boston: Butterworth-Heinemann.

Study and Review Questions

1. Why are crime prevention programs important?
    - A. They offer cost-effective, proactive solutions to security-related issues
    - B. They educate employees to be the eyes and ears of security
    - C. They are easily modified to fit specific situations and issues
    - D. All of the above

2. Which of the following is not a tool used in identifying program topics and developing safety tips?
    - A. Conducting surveys
    - B. Analyzing incident reports
    - C. Addressing seasonal concerns
    - D. Securing computer equipment

3. Which of these is not an example of a problem-oriented program?
    - A. Multi-disciplinary taskforce
    - B. Vehicle "hard target" flyer
    - C. Unattended/unsecured area patrol notice
    - D. Bike patrol

4. Complete the statement, "Crime prevention is..."
    - A. Everyone's responsibility
    - B. Up to security
    - C. Up to the police
    - D. Impossible

Chapter 15

Developing Training Plans and Programs

Scott Buff

OBJECTIVES

After studying this chapter, the student should understand the following:

- The different styles of adult learning
- What is in a training plan
- What a needs assessment is and how it is used
- What performance objectives are and their role in a training program
- What is in a lesson plan packet
- Liability issues pertinent to conducting training

Training is essential to today's healthcare security department. The lack of training has often caused great criticism of the profession. A department's ability, morale, and credibility are all products of proper training. Training is a means toward high-level performance by participants. Training activities help develop a person's abilities to gain knowledge, acquire skills, and employ problem-solving methods.

Training is more than just providing information. Training requires a practical demonstration that each employee has acquired the skill or knowledge related to the job.

Many instances call for training and an educational program to be developed. Employees should be trained at the times noted in the sidebar.

When to Train

- At the start of employment
- When reassigned or transferred to a new position
- At the introduction of new equipment, processes, or procedures
- When performance does not meet standards
- When non-routine tasks must be performed

Adult Learners

Methods to facilitate adult learning have changed greatly in recent years. The art and science of helping adults learn is called andragogy. Andragogy explains the differences between the way adults and children learn. Techniques used to train adults are different than those for children. To design training that meets the needs of your adult learners, you need to (1) be familiar with the principles of adult learning and (2) understand the characteristics of adult learners. Key points about adult learning are summarized in the sidebar on the following page.

Principles of Adult Learning

Adults' needs can be translated into these five learning principles.

- *Relevance:* The information required to be learned must be relevant to the adult's life or particular needs.
- *Self-directed Learning:* Adults are capable of self-direction and see themselves as autonomous.
- *Linked to Experience:* Adults have past experiences. If possible, these previous experiences need to be tapped into as a resource for the learning activity.
- *Practical:* Adults' readiness to learn comes from their desire to influence their lives. They learn best when they see the practical application of what is being taught.
- *Internally Motivated:* Adults are internally motivated. They want to learn new skills to increase job satisfaction.

Characteristics of Adult Learners

Training programs need to incorporate a variety of teaching methods suited to the learning styles and preferences of adults.

Styles of Learning. Every individual has a unique style of learning that determines how he or she learns new information most naturally and effectively. The training should suit all three styles of learning: visual, auditory, and experiential.

- *Visual Learning:* Some adults learn best when they can see the information. They rely on visual aids, such as PowerPoint presentations, flip charts, pictures, and videos. They tend to take lots of notes.
- *Auditory Learning:* These participants learn by hearing information. Lecture, discussion, and repeating information to themselves enables auditory learners to best understand the information. A rule of thumb is to repeat important information three times for retention.
- *Experiential Learning:* Most adults learn best by doing. They prefer to be involved, moving, experiencing, and experimenting. These learners rely on group discussions, practice sessions, and simulations.

Adult Preferences. Adults are valuable resources for the instructor as well as for one another. Their need to understand their own life experiences becomes a motivation to engage in activities and learn. Adults want to take responsibility for their learning and to engage in a learning community, and the learning environment created must reflect this.

- *Responsibility:* Adults, unlike children, do not assume the instructor has the only responsibility for teaching the material. They believe they must take responsibility for their own learning. Adults prefer to have a voice in what is taught, how it is taught, and when it is taught.
- *Learning Community:* Adult learners have a desire to connect and support each other's learning. To address this characteristic, instructors should use students in the teaching (a collaborative approach) and encourage cooperation and communication between participants and the instructor. Allowing participants to set performance objectives and goals and to facilitate a learning activity themselves fosters this.

Applying every principle and characteristic of adult learning is not always feasible. However, knowing them greatly assists in developing the needs assessment, performance objectives, training plan, and lesson plans.

Security's Training Plan

Well before you offer any specific training course, you, and any other managers in the security organization, need to have identified the training needs of security staff. Department management synthesizes this information into a comprehensive training plan for security staff. This chapter uses the term "training plan" to refer to the big-picture document that describes all training for the department; the term "training program," as used in this chapter, refers to training on a specific topic (e.g., a class or course).

The process starts with a big-picture analysis and ends with a detailed lesson plan for each program in the plan. The paragraphs that follow delineate the key steps in developing your department's overall training plan and the specific programs and courses within it. The main elements are these:

- Needs assessment
- Performance objectives
- Training plan
- Lesson plans

Needs Assessment

A needs assessment should be the first step in any overall training plan and in any specific training program. Systematically explore the gaps between the current situation and the desired or necessary situation in relation to the issue in question. Conduct periodic reviews to ensure the training program is still relevant and applicable to your needs.

Current Situation
In your analysis of the current situation, consider the following:

- The present state of skills, knowledge, and the abilities of the employees
- The specific organizational goal, climate, and internal and external constraints

Desired Situation
In your analysis of the desired or necessary situation, focus on the following:

- Necessary standards for change
- Skills, knowledge, and abilities to accomplish these successfully

Identify the desired or necessary conditions for both organizational and personal change. Do not just observe current practices. Distinguish between *actual needs* and *perceived needs or wants*.

Questions to Consider
To facilitate the needs assessment, ask the following questions.

- ***What does the organization/department want or expect from the training?*** Outline official expectations.
- ***What administrative support and materials are readily available?*** Are other sources of help or materials available, or will the creator of the program be responsible for all logistics?
- ***What does the course facilitator know?*** Determine if the skill to conduct this training exists in-house. Will someone need to attend a train-the-trainer course or will a local expert be brought in?
- ***What are the goals and objectives of the training program?*** What changes are desired in the knowledge, skills, and attitudes of the participants? How will we assess whether the goals and objectives have been achieved?

Goals Statements
Each training plan should have clear goals statements that introduce the concepts to be conveyed via training. Explain why this training is occurring.

After your department has completed the needs assessment and the goals statement, the next step is defining each program's performance objectives.

Performance Objectives

The performance objectives, based on the needs assessment and goals statement, should be the central focus in preparing each training program. Performance objectives are the framework for the lesson plan. By clarifying the objectives in the planning phase, you facilitate the selection and design of materials, content, and instructional method. The objectives should also always be clearly explained to program participants so they know what is important.

Types of Performance Objectives

There are basically three types of performance objectives: cognitive, affective, and behavioral. Determine what type of objective(s) each training program should have.

- *Cognitive* performance objectives relate to what the participant will perceive, comprehend, or remember. The participant should receive clear information and develop knowledge.

- *Affective* performance objectives communicate what the participant will feel, value, or become committed to or enthusiastic about. The participant will become sensitized to the issue in question.

- *Behavioral* performance objectives state what the participant will be able to do, perform, demonstrate, use, or explain. The participant will acquire or reinforce skills.

Useful Performance Objectives

Confirm that the performance objectives are consistent with the overall learning goals and with the knowledge and skills of the trainers. To ensure a program's performance objectives are useful, structure them as follows:

- State them in behavioral terms
- State them in clear language
- Make them narrow, specific, and measurable
- Design them to be achievable within the allotted time and in terms of learning resources

Flexibility and adaptability need to be built into the performance objectives. The objectives must empower the trainer to incorporate varied and interactive training techniques. Varying the teaching techniques used throughout the program secures and retains active engagement of participants. The objectives also have to be suitable for evaluating learning results. See the sidebar for guidance on how to write performance objectives.

Chapter 15: Developing Training Plans and Programs

How to Write Performance Objectives

- Begin the objective with a statement of the expected result or task. State what the student will physically be able to accomplish after training (e.g., "After this program, participants will be able to…").

- When defining what measurable result the participants will be able to accomplish, use the appropriate action verb (e.g., identify, write, list, describe, recite, construct, conduct, evaluate, organize, develop, define, apply, illustrate, create, analyze, utilize). Avoid ambiguous or immeasurable words.

- State the condition or circumstance under which the task will occur and include what tools or equipment the participant will be allowed to use.

- State the specific skills being developed and any environmental conditions under which the participant will be expected to perform.

- End the performance objective with the standard. The standard is a measurement of how well the participant performs. The standard must be observable and measurable. Express the standard in terms of speed or time limit, accuracy, quality, or resultant ability. An example of a good standard for a report writing class is this: "After this course, the participant will, with the use of a dictionary, be able to write a report that is clear, concise, accurate, legible, and detailed."

Training Plan

Development and execution of a well-conceived training plan is the foundation upon which a successful training program rests. A training plan can be developed for an entire organization or for a specific unit.

A corporate plan addresses the training needs of an entire organization. The plan may cover a relatively elastic time period of perhaps several years (this is a reflection of a global or overall set of goals).

More common is a training plan specific to a smaller unit within the organization. The plan covers a discrete fiscal or calendar timeframe (this is a reflection of concrete, measurable goals and objectives).

Although there is more than one way to construct a training plan, certain elements need to be considered. The sidebar below outlines the eight major topics that must be addressed in the plan, and the paragraphs that follow detail each.

Contents of a Training Plan

1. Background
2. Current status
3. Mission statement
4. Methods
5. Description of training
6. Performance objectives
7. Implementation
8. Schedule and budget

Background

The training plan should begin with a section providing background. The background section will be predominantly narrative in structure and answer the following:

- Why is a training plan needed?
- Who are the core participants and what is the total number of participants?
- What other factors underline the need for training (e.g., new requirements put upon the organization or department)?

Current Status

The purpose of the current status section is to describe what sort of training has been completed to date. This section needs to be updated each year and referenced against the previous year for comparative purposes. Include the results of the needs assessment. Below are some of the key questions to be answered:

- What type of training has been completed to date?
- Has the training been just-in-time and demand-driven or was there a previous formal training plan?
- If there was a previous training plan, to what extent has it been completed? If factors limited the training, explain them.
- Is there a training budget? What is the budget? How much, if any, has already been spent?

Mission Statement

The mission statement states what you hope to achieve in an overall sense with the training plan. Reaching the overall goal in one to five years would be very challenging. One or several different types of training may be required. You probably need to conduct a number of courses to reach the overall goal.

The overall goal of a training plan differs from course goals and objectives, which tend to be more specific to the training and more limited in scope. Course goals and objectives are also more measurable than the overall goal because participants can assist in assessing whether the goals and objectives have been met.

Methods

The methods section outlines the approaches to training delivery that will be employed. For example, the training plan may extend over two years or five years to instruct all participants in only one course, or a phased approach may be more appropriate. General training may be conducted the first year and more advanced training the following year. The methodology section describes how the overall goal is reached as well as the types of training that will be offered. For example:

- Will the training be via videoconference, materials that participants sign out, online, or a traditional classroom setting?
- Who will participate in the training?
- How many hours will the program require to complete, how many sessions, and over what period of time?

The training methodology should be updated every year as delivery methods are evaluated.

Description of Training

In this section, the training plan becomes more specific, both in terms of deliverables and timeframes. If more than one type of training is to be accomplished, this section is repeated so that each type of training is described.

Goals

The goals section addresses the following:

- What goals are to be achieved from the specific training programs in the plan?
- Who will benefit from this training?

Performance Objectives

Performance objectives, developed as part of the plan, are listed in the training plan.

Implementation

Here, your plan acknowledges what is needed to bring about the training objectives. This section has two parts: how training delivery will be coordinated and what materials are needed.

Coordination. You have to plan how each training program will be delivered. This section notes the coordination activities required for each program.

- What facilities will be used for training?
- What are the dates of the training?
- Is attendance mandatory or voluntary? If voluntary, will there be a registration? How will participants register?

- How will the training be delivered?
- How will the results of the training be evaluated?

The evaluation process is implemented to analyze the delivery outcomes and identify any shortfalls of the training method.

Materials. This section considers and defines material needs, answering the following:
- What materials are needed (e.g., manual, slides, PowerPoint presentation, handouts)?

Schedule and Budget

This section provides sufficient information about the following for each program:

- Date of training
- Method of training
- Cost of training
- Approximate number of participants to be trained

Points to Consider

An Important Framework. Although you must avoid making the plan too complex, recognize that without some kind of framework the exhaustive training efforts your department undertakes may not bear the fruit they should.

Executive Summary. Once you have developed the training plan, you can work on the executive summary. Appearing at the beginning of the training report, the executive summary summarizes key points for the organization's administration, including the following:

- Successes to date
- Challenges ahead
- This year's activities (goals, programs, courses, and planning activities)
- Potential impact on staff and budget for the coming fiscal year

Annual Review. Consider the type of reporting to be done when the annual round of training is completed. Summarizing the information in the training plan is a good place to start. After that, you can flesh out your report with the actual costs and number of participants trained. This information helps form part of your overall evaluation of training.

Lesson Plan Packets

A lesson plan packet needs to be developed for each course being implemented. A lesson plan packet accounts for everything that the instructor and participants must do, from the moment the course starts until it ends. The lesson plan packet consists of the following:

- Cover sheet
- Lesson plan
- Presentation materials
- Participant materials
- Assessment methods

Lesson plan packets may be prepared and provided to the instructor as a set of print materials or as a set of resources accessed via computer.

Cover Sheet

The cover sheet lists the following:

- Course title
- Timeframe or length of the course (normally expressed in hours)
- Date the packet was prepared and dates the packet was reviewed and/or revised
- Person(s) who prepared the packet
- Lead instructor(s) and backup instructor(s)
- Performance objectives

Lesson Plan

The lesson plan consists of the following:

- Main heading containing the course title
- Outline, including introduction, body, and conclusion as well as transitions

- Notes to the instructor that, among other things, assist the instructor in identifying the performance objectives and knowing when to present the presentation materials

Presentation Materials

This section not only provides the presentation materials, but also describes what is needed in the classroom. The following items must be listed:

- *Materials:* Any transparencies, slides, PowerPoint presentations, or other presentation materials to be used are identified and provided. If materials are not physically included in the packet (i.e., they are online or kept in the classroom), the packet notes how the instructor accesses these materials in the learning setting (e.g., by providing an online link or by noting where materials are stored).
- *Equipment:* Items needed to conduct the course, including what is needed to display materials or aid in demonstrations and activities, are listed (e.g., computer, projection screen, white board). As appropriate, provides instructions for course leader on how and when to request equipment and of whom.
- *Setup:* The classroom setup is described or shown, as appropriate. As appropriate, provides instructions for course leader on how and when setup request must be made and to whom.
- *Support Materials:* Any materials the instructor may require and any support materials the instructor may require are listed.

Participant Materials

Participant materials are the workbooks, manuals, handouts, study guides, and so on that need to be distributed and whatever tools or material students must have for the course. These must be included or referenced in the lesson plan packet. As appropriate, the lesson plan states where these materials will be found if they are stored or left in the classroom or on a computer or Intranet.

Assessment Instruments

Finally, the lesson plan packet includes the assessment instruments. All tests and answer keys are provided. Scenario descriptions for performance objectives requiring demonstrations are also provided.

Documentation

The creation of lesson plans ensures standardized coverage of the material in all classes. The lesson plan puts information in logical order and guarantees that performance objectives are met. The lesson plan packet allows a substitute instructor to adequately present the lesson and can boost the confidence of all instructors.

Be sure that the lesson plan is always used, whether the course is run by the intended instructor or a substitute. As the course progresses, check off all points covered and sign and date the lesson plan. This verifies that the information was covered and is invaluable if a liability case ensues. As a record of instruction, the lesson plan greatly aids in liability protection.

Training must document two things: (1) what was trained and (2) who was trained. Litigation may put the organization and trainers in an adverse position unless you can show that the employee's actions were inconsistent with documented training.

Liability Issues

Organizations have an obligation to train their employees for the routine tasks that they face on the job. If, foreseeably, an employee may be confronted with a duty that may result in the harm of another person, the employer must provide training. The training must teach the employee how to conduct that task in a manner consistent with generally accepted practices and reasonable by legal standards. Training is a contribution toward proper performance. Unfortunately, many organizations implement training to avoid, or in response to, litigation rather than to promote high-level performance. Failure-to-train cases are becoming more prevalent.

Failure-to-train cases are established in two ways. The first way is to show lack of training in an area where the need for training is obvious (e.g., a security officer untrained in proper baton techniques uses a baton on someone). A second way is to show a pattern of conduct by employees that would put the organization on notice and the organization then failed to respond with training. However, if a reasonable person would know the proper response to a situation without training, the organization had no duty to train.

One legal precedent in failure to train is *City of Canton Ohio v. Harris*. The Supreme Court stated that "inadequate training may give rise to 42 U.S.C., section 1983 liability when it is deliberately indifferent to the rights of the city's inhabitants and actually causes the plaintiff's injury." As one example of deliberately inadequate training, the Court enumerated "instances in which the need for more or different training is obvious and the inadequacy is likely to result in the violation of constitutional rights."

Areas to Train

When considering the areas to train, a department can apply a simple three-part test:

1. The department must know to an ethical certainty that its officers will confront a given situation.
2. The officer will be faced with a difficult duty that appropriate training will make less problematic (or a history exists of the department's officers mis-handling similar situations).
3. A wrong choice by the officer will likely cause the deprivation of a person's rights or cause unjust harm.

Direct and Vicarious Liability

The two types of liability prudent for consideration when developing training are direct liability and vicarious liability.

Direct Liability. Direct liability is the legal obligation incurred by the instructor and/or organization directly through the training function when negligent acts or omissions results in bodily injury and/or property damage or destruction to another party and there are no intervening circumstances.

Vicarious Liability. Vicarious liability is a form of strict, secondary liability that arises under the common law doctrine of *respondeat superior* (Latin for "let the master answer"). Under this theory of law, an employer is responsible for employee actions performed within the course of the employment. The vicarious liabilities of consideration for the organization are these:

- Negligent retention
- Negligent assignment
- Negligent supervision

Instructors must always cautiously think about being neglectful in failure to train, course preparation, instruction, and documentation. See chapter 9 for more on liability and negligence.

Conclusion

Many instances call for training and educational programs to be developed. A department's ability to successfully research and implement these training programs promotes higher levels of competency and professionalism.

As a supervisor, you need to understand how to develop a training plan and training programs. This involves conducting a needs assessment, defining performance objectives, and developing training plans and lesson plan packets.

As well, you must understand the liabilities associated with training and what the lack of training can mean to an organization. Understanding the liability issues is of utmost importance.

Not only should you be able to develop a training plan and programs, but you should also be able to effectively present the plan to the organization's administration.

Bibliography

City of Canton Ohio v. Harris, 489 U.S. 378, S. Ct. 1197 (1989).

Hornburg, J. 2005. The Lesson Plan Tool Kit (handout distributed at the International Law Enforcement Educators and Trainers Association 2005 International Training Conference, Chicago, Illinois).

Ryan, J. 2006 Aug. Legal/liability issues in the training function. Indianapolis: Public Agency Training Council. On the Internet: http://patc.com/weeklyarticles/liabilitytraining.shtml. Accessed 28 Mar 2007.

Wikipedia. http://en.wikipedia.org/wiki/Andragogy. Accessed 24 Mar 2007.

Study and Review Questions

1. What is the first step in developing a training program?

    A. Developing performance objectives

    B. Conducting a needs assessment

    C. Creating a lesson plan packet

    D. Crafting a training plan

2. When writing performance objectives, which of the following would not be an appropriate verb to use?

    A. Apply

    B. Construct

    C. Evaluate

    D. Know

3. What training-related document describes the current status of training?

    A. Lesson plan packet

    B. Needs assessment

    C. Training plan

    D. Performance objectives

4. Why should training be implemented?

    A. To promote high-level performance

    B. To avoid, or in response to, litigation

    C. To build-in overtime

    D. To spend excess budget

5. When considering an area to train, what question should the department ask?

    A. Are there certain situations that the department has a history of mis-handling?

    B. Will the wrong choice in a given situation be likely to deprive a person of his or her rights or cause unjust harm?

    C. Does the department know to a moral certainty that its officers will be involved in a particular situation?

    D. All of the above

Chapter 16
Security Operations

Stuart G. Fletcher, CHPA, CPP, MBA

OBJECTIVES

After studying this chapter, the student should understand the following:

- How the management reporting structure affects the supervisor's level of participation in a healthcare security program
- How to better maintain an effective security operations program
- The supervisor's responsibilities in monitoring day-to-day operations
- Weekly responsibilities of the supervisor
- Monthly responsibilities of the supervisor
- How dedication to ongoing personal and professional growth contributes to effectiveness
- Importance of fairness and equality in effective supervision

As a security supervisor, you are responsible for your department's daily operations in the healthcare facility. Depending on the style and personality of the person to whom you report (your direct report), you may find yourself responsible for more or less of the program than is described in this chapter.

In this chapter, elements come together from throughout this book. This chapter helps you understand why a supervisor needs to know so many facets of management and leadership.

The supervisor is a critical factor in security's daily operation. You must recognize your level of involvement in the security program. You need to know everything going on in the security department as well as what is happening throughout the facility. You cannot acquire this information by sitting all day in your office reading reports and answering phone calls. Although reading reports and performing clerical work are elements of the job, these tasks should take an hour or two, not the entire workday, to complete.

Be visible to staff in the facility and to the security officers. As you walk around the facility, make your presence known. Doing so enables you to collect useful information and data.

Supervisors speak for and are spoken to about department issues. You must be both an effective spokesperson and gatherer of information. Talk with employees from various departments about their security concerns. This helps educate the staff. This contact also brings you valuable information on situations not reported via security incident reports. This information can be a key factor when deciding how to assign security staff to patrol responsibilities.

Understanding the Reporting Hierarchy

Security supervisors may report to the head of the security department or a manager of another department in the healthcare organization. Supervisors who are employees of a contracted security firm have dual reporting responsibilities: to someone at the security firm and someone at the healthcare facility. The paragraphs that follow discuss aspects of each situation.

Reporting to an In-house Security Manager or Director

Some security supervisors report to the healthcare organization's security manager. In this situation, your level of participation depends on how "hands on" your manager is.

Usually, the supervisor handles day-to-day operations, and the manager handles administrative aspects of the department. The manager attends meetings, makes policy changes, reviews the overall budget and operation, and handles other administrative duties. The supervisor ensures patrols are conducted correctly and effectively, security's response to special situations such as escorts is appropriate, and reports are being handled and written in a timely manner. The supervisor ensures that every security officer is correctly and aptly trained for the job responsibilities specific to each shift and each day of the week.

Reporting to a Facilities Manager or Other In-house Manager

Some security supervisors report to the facilities manager or to another manager in the healthcare organization—someone outside the security department. In this situation, you have more responsibility than if you had a manager within the security department.

In this type of arrangement, you must know more about legal aspects and security operations so you can effectively run the department. You must know if the department is legally able to carry out requests made of it.

For example, you may be asked to supply security staff at a local high school for a basketball game sponsored by your institution. In some jurisdictions, in-house security officers may only work on property owned by the institution; there, you would have to decline the request for staff to work at a school.

Reporting to a Contract Service and an In-house Manager

Some security supervisors are not employees of the healthcare organization. Rather, they are employees of a security company contracted to provide security services for the healthcare organization. Such supervisors report to a field supervisor and an office manager of their employer (the security company) as well as to a manager within the healthcare organization.

In this situation, you must understand that although you are conducting a service for the healthcare facility at which you work, your allegiance must be to the company that employs you. This balance is difficult to maintain. Supervisors in this situation often may become close with the client. The relationship must never compromise the contract services. If you do what the healthcare organization wants and do not follow your company's rules, regulations, and contract, your actions may put the healthcare organization, your company, and you in a legally compromising situation.

The best part of having a contract services relationship is that you have many experienced security resources within the agency to use when you need help or advice. When the client asks you to do something and you are not sure if it is within your job responsibilities, contact your firm for input. The firm's staff will help you explain to the client why something can or cannot be done. The firm may even send an office representative to smooth things with the client to keep you out of the picture.

Maintaining Effective Security Operations

As a supervisor, you are the person in the middle. You represent the security administration to security officers, and you represent the security officers to security administration.

To be a successful supervisor, you must acknowledge and exhibit basic leadership qualities, explains Russell Colling in *Hospital and Healthcare Security* (Colling 2001, p. 149). Leaders, notes Colling, are expected to do the following:

- Set a good example; motivate subordinates by showing them what is expected

- Do not insist on agreement with everything you do or say
- Make allowances for inexperience and unintentional mistakes
- Be considerate of the personal needs of the officers, but understand that the needs of the organization must be given highest priority
- Give ground on small items, but never compromise on principles
- See those you supervise and be seen by them
- Have the courage to make objective decisions even when you know the decisions are not popular

In short, you must "accept ownership of your responsibility as a supervisor," writes Colling. "Successful leadership is characterized by involvement, participation, and commitment. Thus, supervisory responsibility is not for everyone" (Colling 2001, p. 149).

Deploying Resources

Deployment of security officers is an important element in staffing a security program. Optimally, staffing ratios increase at peak times (e.g., at times when a high number of incidents typically occur and at shift changes for facility staff, when requests for personal escorts rise sharply). However, in the reality of our times and with the financial constraints in the healthcare industry, security usually functions with minimal staffing. That is one reason you must help ensure that patrols are not predictably routine. Predictability lets the criminal element know exactly when they can and cannot strike.

Encourage officers to be proactive. Officers must constantly look at their surroundings for potential problems, rather than merely walk with tunnel vision toward the next badging station. During shift changes, post security officers at known exits for employees. If auto thefts increase in a certain parking lot, increase the number of patrols there. Know what is going on throughout the facility so you can best deploy resources—the security officers.

In handing out assignments, make sure that the officers are aware of their responsibilities within each of the tasks. To do this, you must be able to handle any task that the officers may handle—on all three shifts, seven days a week. Whether the task is assigning response priorities of the dispatcher or responding to a stat call, you need to know every aspect before you can teach the job function to others.

A Supervisor's Day-to-day Responsibilities

Ensuring that your direct report and the hospital risk manager are aware of all security incidents reported within the healthcare facility is your responsibility. With your fingers on the pulse of the hospital's activity, you are an integral part of the security management program. Daily responsibilities vary, depending on the facility as well as personalities and management styles. Here are examples of what you may handle on a daily, and ongoing, basis:

- Ensure that each member of the department is an active public relations/customer service officer
- Ensure adequate coverage for daily operations
- Give staff positive reinforcement each day
- Proactively look for new or better ways of doings things; correct problems before they become issues
- Handle complaints in a positive manner
- Handle disciplinary problems as necessary, make your direct report aware of any disciplinary actions in the department, and jointly handle any terminations with your direct report
- Make sure the workload is evenly distributed among all staff
- Enforce policy through example
- Meet daily, weekly, or as needed with your direct report to keep communications open and keep both parties informed of all upcoming changes
- If you are a contract supervisor, report events and situations to your contract firm

as well as to the healthcare organization (except exclusively contract-services issues)

- Bring problems and possible solutions to your direct report and/or contract firm when you are not sure which course of action to take; seek a mutually acceptable course of action

A Supervisor's Weekly Responsibilities

Stay on top of all the daily and weekly responsibilities you are assigned. Supervisors can quickly fall behind by not handling job duties as intended. Some tasks, such as payroll, require daily and weekly action. Weekly responsibilities vary, depending on the facility as well as personalities and management styles. Here are examples of what you may handle on a weekly, and ongoing, basis:

- *Payroll:* Monitor daily and post weekly
- *Schedule:* Develop a biweekly schedule, wisely using staff to minimize overtime and provide optimal coverage at key times
- *Uniforms:* Authorize with direct report's signature, when applicable
- *Proactive Management:* Correct what is wrong instead of merely reporting it to management

A Supervisor's Monthly Responsibilities

Do not make the mistake of thinking that monthly responsibilities are less important than daily or weekly ones. Routinely evaluate all aspects of the security department for effectiveness. Training may seem like another compliance issue, but think how much more valuable your officers become as they increase their job knowledge. Under your mentoring and training, shift leads may be able to pick up some of your less critical responsibilities. This gives you more time for other job demands.

When staff members are empowered with these new responsibilities, they grow professionally and become a more valuable asset—to both you and the organization. If you receive a promotion to a managerial position, you will have some excellent internal candidates to choose from for your second-in-command.

Expect to handle the following items, at a minimum, on a monthly basis. Depending on personalities and management styles, your monthly responsibilities may include the following:

- Ensure full compliance with safety, security, and other training requirements.
- Complete all evaluations in a timely manner, and make sure other shift leads are doing the same.
- Review department policies, procedures, and guidelines to see if anything that is occurring is not addressed. Work with management to get this corrected.
- Refer to your job description for more direction and detailed information.
- Have team meetings with the other security supervisors to evaluate the needs of the department.
- Based on the information gained in the supervisors' meetings, schedule department meetings, and training sessions identified as appropriate.
- Your direct report and contract service firm are valuable resources. Do not be afraid to admit you do not know something or that you need help from them; that is why they are there.

Valuing Personal Growth

By seeking personal growth in the supervisory position, you stay on the cutting edge of management. Look for opportunities among the following:

- *Professional Certification:* Take more programs like this one. Obtain the Certified Healthcare Protection Administrator (CHPA) designation.
- *Management Training:* Take courses offered by your employer and from local colleges and adult education programs.
- *Professional Associations:* Whenever possible, go to conferences and events from related professional organizations, such as the IAHSS and ASIS International. Become an active member in both organizations. As you learn more about managing and leadership, you become more confident and willing to mentor and train those around you.
- *Departmental Issues:* In addition to formal education, find growth within your department that will enrich your interest in the position. This increases your value to the security department, healthcare organization, and contract service.

The sidebar lists some activities you may be able to assume for your department. Do not limit yourself to these. As a supervisor, you know what needs to be done, what needs to be changed, and what needs to be instituted. Always have the approval of your direct report or contract firm; do not do these things on your own. The only exception would be if you have earned your manager's respect and trust and been given that latitude of initiative.

Opportunities and Goals for Supervisors' Personal and Professional Growth

- Volunteer to write or revise a policy
- Complete the purge of archives
- Become proficient on computerized systems for writing incident reports
- Learn the camera system and recording/reviewing capabilities well enough to teach others
- Create a department orientation packet
- Learn to make employee identification badges
- Learn to operate the door access system
- Take relevant computer classes to improve your knowledge
- Test panic alarms and emergency phones monthly, and submit that information to your direct report monthly
- Be timely in submitting monthly reports
- Ensure fire extinguisher inspections are timely and complete
- Periodically test emergency response of the department (response time to a stat call)
- Institute a proactive theft deterrent program

Ensuring Fairness and Equality

A supervisor must assume many responsibilities. Accepting this role means you are both willing to accept and capable of handling the responsibilities of this position. You must be firm when enforcing the institution's policies and fair about enforcing them with everyone equally.

You cannot play favorites. Despite personality differences, you must treat each subordinate officer equally, with courtesy and respect. Bullying and intimidating to achieve respect misses the mark. You must earn respect from those above you as well as those reporting to you. Treat everyone as you would like to be treated: although almost every supervisory book written advises this, this principle is one of the first things many supervisors seem to forget. To be a professional, you must act like a professional.

This does not mean you lack compassion for your staff. Always remember that your officers are people, just like you. They have feelings, and they have personal lives that can slip over into their work lives. Good supervisors are "people persons." They like helping and nurturing people. They enjoy mentoring and teaching and watching their staff grow within their positions and as people. People persons enjoy this work because they care for people and want to help them in every way.

Look at how you treat people from their perspective, not yours. See how your staff perceives you. Sometimes this assessment can be shocking. Once you overcome your initial disbelief, seek out ways to better yourself as a person and as a supervisor. Ask others what they think you should improve to become better at what you do. You may be surprised at how much their feedback, when taken in a positive vein, helps you discover and correct your faults.

Conclusion

A supervisor must assume many responsibilities. Confirm that you are willing to accept and capable of handling these responsibilities.

The reporting method used at your institution helps dictate your level of participation in the security program. Reporting to someone with knowledge about security allows you to concentrate more on daily activities of the department and less on administrative aspects. When working for a contract firm, you report to a manager at the healthcare facility, but must remain loyal to your employer, the contract firm.

Maintaining an effective security operations program has a lot to do with knowing what is actually going on at the hospital. This extends well beyond knowing what is being reported in incident reports. Besides ensuring proper training for all officers, you have daily, weekly, and monthly responsibilities to fulfill. Commit yourself to being timely with these.

Recognize also that despite personality differences, you must treat each subordinate fairly and equally, with courtesy and respect. Look at how you treat each person through that person's eyes, not through your own.

The key to success and personal satisfaction in supervision is understanding that the position requires continual growth. Personal and professional growth can take place in many ways—for example, through classes and certifications and via professional memberships and networking with other security professionals. Some of the best growth may come from mentoring and training others.

Acknowledgment

The author thanks Joel Wiesner, CHPA, of Fontana, California, for editing this manuscript.

Bibliography

Colling, R. L. 2001. *Hospital and Healthcare Security*, 4th ed. Boston: Butterworth-Heinemann.

Study and Review Questions

1. Supervisors typically are responsible for what type of operations of the security department?

    A. Day-to-day

    B. Administrative

    C. Personnel

    D. Risk management

2. Which of the following is not a basic leadership quality?

    A. Set a good example

    B. Be visible

    C. Insist on agreement with everything

    D. Make objective decisions

3. Which of the following is not a way to enhance your professional growth in the organization?

    A. Learn to make identification badges

    B. Rely on vendor to operate the door access system

    C. Ensure reports are turned in on time

    D. Learn the camera system

4. Which of the following is important to maintain an effective security operation?

    A. Rely only on what is being reported through security incident reports

    B. Know what is actually going on and what is being reported

    C. Rely only on what is actually going on

    D. Rely on facility incident reports

5. Which of the following is not a component of a proactive patrol?

    A. Random times of patrol

    B. Constantly looking for potential problems

    C. Random routes of patrol

    D. Predictable patterns

Chapter 17

Planning for Emergency Management and Response

Stephen W. Gaunt, MBA, CHPA

OBJECTIVES

After studying this chapter, the student should understand the following:

- Emergency and disaster declaration process
- The Hospital Incident Command System
- The security supervisor's role during a disaster or emergency

---

A mass casualty or disaster incident occurs when any large number of casualties is produced in a relatively short period of time, usually resulting from a single incident (e.g., terrorist attack, hurricane, earthquake, flood, major traffic accident, airplane crash) that exceeds the ability of community resources and healthcare to respond or treat the victims. An emergency is an event that causes an influx of patients out of the ordinary scope but is within the abilities of the facility.

Since 1953, the Federal Emergency Management Agency (FEMA) has recorded 1706 federally declared major disasters. The following statistics give a sense of when and how often disaster has struck (FEMA 2007):

- Each year in the United States, on average, 31 major disasters are declared
- 2004 was the year with the single highest yearly total (68); 1958 had the lowest number of disasters (7)
- Since 1953, Texas has the highest yearly cumulative total of declared disasters (79), followed by California (72), Florida (59), and Wyoming, Utah, Rhode Island, and the District of Columbia (with 7 each)
- Halfway through 2007, six emergencies had been declared for the year, involving snow, severe winter storms, and flooding in five states

To effectively respond to major disasters and emergencies, healthcare organizations throughout the United States must invest financial resources, personnel, time, and training to ensure adequate preparations are in place. The 1706 major disasters and recent events such as the September 11, 2001 terrorism attack, the 2004 Severe Acute Respiratory Syndrome (SARS) outbreak, and the 2006 Gulf Coast hurricanes (Katrina, Wilma, and Rita) all demonstrate the importance of preparedness. These major disasters identified the need for healthcare organizations to be self-sustaining and to be prepared to receive little or no immediate assistance from the community, state, or federal resources. During these disasters, the public looked to healthcare institutions and the medical community to provide refuge, shelter, food, medical care, and security. When the community infrastructure collapses, healthcare facilities must continue to be self-sustaining. They must also be surviving entities unto themselves. A healthcare facility should be prepared to support itself in the early days of a disaster. The healthcare facility should be able to provide ongoing medical care, evacuations when necessary, facility protection, and recovery with little or no help from the government.

The Process of Declaring an Emergency or Disaster

Emergency Declaration

Declaring an emergency usually follows these steps:

1. *Notification:* Healthcare facility receives notification that it will be receiving an influx of patients.
2. *Verification:* Facility verifies ability to provide care to the estimated influx with existing staff and gears up to handle the influx.

Disaster Declaration

Declaring a major disaster usually follows these steps:

1. *Local government responds,* supplemented by neighboring communities and volunteer agencies. The mayor, city council, or county executive may declare a state of emergency. If overwhelmed, local government turns to the state for assistance.
2. *States respond* with state resources, such as the National Guard and state agencies.
3. *Damage assessment* by local, state, and volunteer organizations determines losses and recovery needs.
4. *A major disaster declaration* is requested by the governor, based on the damage assessment, and an agreement is made to commit state funds and resources to the long-term recovery.
5. *FEMA evaluates* the request and recommends action to the White House based on the disaster, the local community, and the state's ability to recover.
6. *The President of the United States approves* the request or the FEMA informs the governor the request has been denied. This decision process could take a few hours or several weeks depending on the nature of the disaster.

The Healthcare Institution's Response

Your facility's disaster plan may contain benchmarks that would automatically trigger activation of the emergency response plan independently of any declaration by a local, state, or federal agency. Following Hurricane Katrina in 2006, many healthcare facilities have written into their plans to automatically activate the disaster plan 24 to 48 hours before landfall of any major hurricane. In states where blizzards are frequent, healthcare facilities have written their plans to automatically activate when the prediction for snow exceeds 12 to 18 inches.

As a security supervisor, you must be fully familiar with your facility's disaster preparedness plan and what mechanism triggers activation of the plan. During off shifts or in the absence of the security manager, you may be asked to provide input to the administrator on call or the nursing supervisor on when to activate the plan.

Improving Disaster and Emergency Response

After a disaster or emergency, most agencies and hospitals conduct debriefing sessions. The aim is to identify failures or areas needing improvement in the disaster or emergency response process. Throughout reviews by various agencies, common failures or weakness have been identified in the response process:

- Inadequate communication because of conflicting terminology or inefficient or improper use of technology, which results in responding agencies failing to communicate effectively

- Lack of a standardized management structure that would allow integration, command and control, and workload efficiency

- Lack of personnel accountability
- Lack of a systematic planning process

The Hospital Incident Command System

As a result of these and other failures, disasters of all sizes and types were often managed inappropriately, resulting in health and safety risks to responders, delay of medical care to victims, ineffective resource use, and economic losses. To meet these challenges, the Hospital Incident Command System (HICS) is designed to do the following:

- Be usable for managing all emergencies or unplanned disasters, of any type or size, by establishing a clear chain of command
- Allow personnel from different agencies or departments to be integrated into a common structure
- Provide needed logistical and administrative support to operational personnel
- Ensure key functions are covered and eliminate duplication

The HICS is a management system. The primary beneficiaries of this system are the healthcare organization's disaster response team, physicians, nurses, and operational and administrative personnel. The HICS system is designed to reduce roles and title confusion.

The HICS was created by a team of individuals after the government mandated that facilities receiving funds from the Health Resources and Services Administration (HRSA) of the US Department of Health and Human Services use the National Incident Management System (NIMS). The Hospital Emergency Incident Command System (HEICS) was changed to the HICS version to comply with the federal mandate. The HICS follows the NIMS and meets the federal requirements. The HICS focuses on healthcare response and incorporates the requirements that are specific to healthcare.

The Incident Commander

Each disaster or incident is managed by the Incident Commander. This position is always activated regardless of the size of the disaster. The Incident Commander sets the objectives, devises strategies and priorities, and maintains overall responsibility for managing the disaster. Depending on the assistance the Incident Commander requires, the Incident Commander may assign additional duties to Section Chiefs for the following areas:

- Operations
- Planning
- Logistics
- Finance/Administration

The Incident Commander may be able to accomplish all five management functions alone on small-scale disasters, but on larger incidents effective management may require the Incident Commander to establish one or more of the functions.

Security Branch Director

As a security supervisor, you may be appointed as the Security Branch Director reporting to the Operations Chief, depending on the scope of the disaster and at the discretion of the Incident Commander or Operations Chief. As such, you should review the Security Services Leader job description for the HICS. Your responsibilities will include, but not be limited to, the items noted in the sidebar on the following page.

Responsibilities of the Security Services Leader

When appointed to be a HICS Security Services Leader in a disaster response, you must consider the need for the following:

- Emergency lockdown
- Security/bomb sweep of designated areas
- Providing urgent security-related information to all personnel
- The need for security personnel to use personal protective equipment
- Removing unauthorized personnel from restricted areas
- Security to sensitive areas
- Controlling the media
- Re-routing of ambulance entry and exit
- Patrol of parking and shipping areas
- Traffic control
- Participating in briefings and meetings as requested
- Documenting all communications (internal and external)
- Ensuring disaster victims' valuable and personal belongings are secured
- Securing any items of evidence
- Coordinating activities with local law enforcement or supporting agencies

Emergency Preparedness Plans

Your organization's emergency preparedness efforts are influenced by a number of regulating agencies and laws, including those listed in the table.

Key Regulatory Agencies and Laws Guiding Emergency Preparedness

The Joint Commission	Environment of Care Standards (EC.4.20)
Occupational Safety and Health Administration (OSHA)	Best practices for hospital-based first receivers of victims from mass casualty incidents involving the release of hazardous substances 29 CFR Part 1910: Hazardous materials, personal protective equipment, and toxic and hazardous substances 29 CFR 1910-120: OSHA hazardous waste operations and emergency response (HAZWOPER)
Emergency Medical Treatment and Active Labor Act (EMTALA)	Anyone presenting to the emergency department is entitled to receive medical care
Health Insurance Portability and Accountability Act of 1996 (HIPAA, Title II)	Personal information is protected at all times
FEMA	
Department of Health (for the state)	

As a security supervisor responsible for implementing the security management portion of the emergency response plan during a disaster, you must regularly investigate for changes in the standards and regulations of these agencies and laws to keep abreast of newly published materials or requirements. You can accomplish this through a combination of resources:

- Attend education seminars
- Conduct Internet searches
- Review documents
- Frequently hold conversations with security supervisors from other healthcare organizations
- Attend Office of Emergency Management (OEM) meetings in your community

Emergency Management Process

Healthcare organizations have emergency management committees or response teams usually consisting of representatives from safety, security, facilities management, clinical staff, infection control, ancillary staff, and the organization's leadership. As a security supervisor, you have major responsibilities in the success of your institution's disaster planning process. Security is a key element in any organization's emergency management process. The emergency management process is made up of the following:

- Hazard vulnerability analysis
- Emergency management/disaster plan
- Drills

Hazard Vulnerability Analysis

The vulnerability analysis is designed to identify risks that directly affect the healthcare facility. All healthcare facilities are subject to internal failures (e.g., utility failures, fire, communication failures, medical gas disruption, labor disruption). A facility may also be vulnerable based on its location. The healthcare facility has a responsibility to identify the vulnerabilities in its region (e.g., thunderstorms, earthquakes). See the table on this page for examples.

Examples of Disaster Risks Based on Location

Region	Risk
Alaska California	Earthquakes and forest fires
Alabama Florida Louisiana Mississippi Texas	Hurricanes
Hawaii Oregon Washington 　(the state)	Volcanos
Kansas Oklahoma	Tornados
New York (the state) Washington, DC	Terrorist attacks and electrical grid failures (blackouts)

Plans and Drills

Healthcare facilities should *review* their emergency/disaster plans at least annually. The plans, however, should be *amended* as needed; that is, whenever changes that could affect their effectiveness occur within the organization or community. Healthcare facilities are required to *test* their emergency management/disaster plan at least twice a year, either in response to an actual emergency or in a planned exercise.

One of the exercises should be a community-wide drill involving outside community support services (e.g., OEM, police, fire, ambulance, medical corps). An exercise maybe a tabletop session if it is in addition to the two functional exercises. Tabletop exercises do not count as planned exercises. For example, the facility may participate in a regional exercise sponsored by a federal, state, or county agency planning for a regional mass casualty scenario.

Drills should be designed to test the facility's ability to treat patients and mass casualties (surge capacity) at a level above normal operating conditions.

Plan, Do, Act, Check

The emergency management process can be defined by the Plan, Do, Act, Check (PDAC) process. Its steps are outlined in the table. The Joint Commission defines the PDAC process as a plan that provides for continual improvement in the emergency and disaster response process.

Emergency Management: The PDAC Process

PLAN
• Hazard vulnerability analysis
• Emergency management plan
• Multi-disciplinary involvement
• Community collaboration
• Orientation/competency/training
• Communication/information systems

DO
• Mutual aid agreements/memorandums
• Logistics
• Patient information management
• Equipment/supplies
• Patient care management
• Alternative site(s)
• Staffing
• Facility
• Utilities
• Infection control
• Security
• Finance

ACT
• Staff knowledge and training
• Emergency items
• Supplies
• Equipment
• Personal protective equipment
• Decontamination process
• Building mitigation features
• Information management provisions
• Memorandums of understanding (MOUs)

CHECK
• Critique
• Pre-established evaluation tool
• Performance measures
• Use of non-participating observers
• Identify lessons learned
• Identify strengths and weaknesses
• Identify improvements
• Incorporate changes into current plan

Security Supervisor's Role During a Disaster

As a security supervisor, you must read about, understand, and be competent in your role in the emergency management plan. You need to understand expectations and functions assigned during a disaster by the Incident Commander. You also need to know the full role of security and what you need for resources to fulfill the security requirements on campus.

Support and Consultation

In accordance with HICS protocol, the security supervisor or designee provides direct support and consultation to the Incident Commander in the following areas:

- Crowd control
- Media control
- Traffic control
- Access control at points of entry for employees, patients, visitors, and professional staff

As a subject matter expert in this role, you serve the Incident Commander by providing sound judgment, information, guidance, direction, advice, and response to security matters.

Staffing

In addition, during a disaster or drill, you are responsible for the following:

- Independently analyzing and prioritizing security officer assignments
- Developing work plans
- Developing schedules
- Supervising security officers

You need to think through emerging crises quickly and make independent decisions regarding the commitment of staffing. Based on your judgment and consultation with the Incident Commander, you should have the responsibility and authority to increase security staffing based on the disaster's magnitude.

Liaison

As well, you should be the liaison with outside law enforcement agencies and other disaster team members.

Evaluation

At the conclusion of the incident response or during the disaster mitigation process, you should take part in the critique of the response to the emergency or disaster. Here, the focus is on providing recommendations for improvement. Topics you should address are these:

- Report on security's response, including resources and time
- Results, in measurable terms, of security staff's performance in meeting the goals and objectives of the disaster response
- Presenting pertinent data on the incident (i.e., number of patients, number of media)
- Consequences resulting from errors that may have led to loss of life, property damage, wasted financial resources, or reduced effectiveness of interactions with local or state agencies

Conclusion

Disaster can be unpredictable and strike without warning. You and your staff must be ready at all times to respond to the institution's needs at a time of crisis. Although standards and regulations play an important role in preparing a healthcare facility for a disaster or emergency, experience dictates that an educated, motivated, equipped, and highly trained staff is essential to any healthcare organization's disaster response. The security staff is a vital service in the healthcare organization—it cannot fail during a disaster. You must ensure that your staff is trained on every aspect of security's role during a disaster and that your staff remains competent.

During a disaster response, you must be committed to the well-being of the community and safety within the facility. You must place the needs of patients above your own. The community expects nothing less than a total effort from their local healthcare institutions. This may be at the expense of the safety or security of your own family, who could also be victims during the disaster. As a supervisor, you must lead the security officers by example. If you fail in responding to the needs of your institution during a disaster, how can you expect your officers to respond as needed?

As a security supervisor, you are entrusted with the lives, safety, and security not only of the medical staff, but also of the patients and victims of a disaster. Plans must be made for your staff and facility to operate independently of any outside assistance for a period of time that could be several days.

As made clear in Hurricane Katrina and the devastation suffered by the New Orleans healthcare community, the role and responsibility of the security supervisor and security staff is vital. The emergency management process requires you to Plan, Do, Act, and Check to ensure your staff is up to the challenges required of healthcare security during a disaster. Failure can result in the loss of life.

Bibliography

Federal disaster declarations. Last modified 3 Jul 2007. On the Internet: www.fema.gov/news/disasters.fema#em. Washington, DC: Federal Emergency Management Agency. Accessed 5 Jul 2007.

Hospital Incident Command System Guidebook. Aug 2006. Sacramento: California Emergency Medical Services Authority. On the Internet: www.emsa.ca.gov/hics/hics.asp. Accessed 21 Jun 2007.

2007 Hospital Accreditation Standards. 2007. Oakbrook Terrace, Ill: The Joint Commission.

Hospitals and Community Emergency Response—What You Need to Know (OSHA 3152). 1997. Washington DC: US Department of Labor Occupational Safety & Health Administration.

Study and Review Questions

1. The HICS is designed to do what?

    A. Improve the hospital's command structure during a crisis, so that it corresponds to other emergency response agencies

    B. Allow the Incident Commander to document the security supervisor's annual Disaster Management Training

    C. Justify the Transportation Officer Chief's position

    D. Be used only when a major disaster or emergency is declared by the FEMA

2. The Joint Commission permits tabletop exercises to count as an emergency preparedness drill under which condition?

    A. Internal disaster exercise involving a simulated utility failure

    B. External disaster exercise involving the local ambulance corps and Boy Scouts as mock patients

    C. Community-wide exercise sponsored by a federal, state, or local agency

    D. Additional drill above the two required

3. During an emergency preparedness exercise or drill, the security supervisor is responsible for what?

    A. Working in a vacuum and not part of the HICS process

    B. Thinking through the emerging crises quickly and making independent decisions regarding the commitment of security staffing

    C. Issuing orders to the medical staff concerning patient medical assessments

    D. Testing the facility's electrical generator to ensure an adequate level of electricity

4. A responsibility of the security supervisor in the emergency management process can be defined as which of these?

    A. Check, Act, Do, Plan (CADP)

    B. Advise the Incident Commander on local media capabilities

    C. Report to the Logistics Chief

    D. Ensure security staff is trained in the emergency management process and understands its assigned roles during a disaster

5. Which of these is an element of disaster mitigation?

    A. Ensure a disaster never happens

    B. Educate staff members on their disaster responsibilities

    C. Minimize the economic impact resulting from the disaster and return the facility to full operations as quickly as possible

    D. Ensure the healthcare organization's insurance premiums are paid

Chapter 18

Supervisor Development

Evelyn Meserve, CHPA

OBJECTIVES

After studying this chapter, the student should understand the following:

- The reason supervisors must not become complacent
- The importance of development tools
- How helping others grow helps the supervisor grow
- Development has many facets
- Development never stops

This chapter builds on chapter 8, Self-Improvement. That chapter, like this one, emphasizes that supervisors must continue to grow and advance in their profession and their position. Allowing yourself to become stagnant or complacent stops you from succeeding. One of the keys in growing as a supervisor is finding the tools to further your personal and professional development and then knowing how to use them and build from them.

If you help others grow in their profession, do you grow with them? Of course, it is a natural progression. We learn in a multitude of ways:

- By helping others
- By mentoring
- By structured learning
- By informal learning

Exploring all these avenues is important. Do not close the door to possibilities.

Tools to Build a Strong Life

According to Marcus Buckingham and Donald O. Clifton, in their book *Now, Discover Your Strengths*, you need three revolutionary tools to build a strong life:

- Understanding how to distinguish your natural talents from things you can learn
- A system to identify your dominant talents
- A common language to describe your talents

How can these three tools help you build a stronger life? If you employ these tools, you are able to learn more about yourself and become comfortable with who you are. We all have strengths and weaknesses; thus, the key to development is knowing how to use them to our advantage and preventing them from overcoming us.

Each facet of character building is different. You need to understand how things affect you. For example, how would you define talents? Talents are what you are blessed with, but your talents are strengthened as you grow. How would you define knowledge? Knowledge is the information, methods, and what you have learned during your life. Finally, how would you define skills? Skills are components of an action. Combine the three—talents, knowledge, and skill—and you have the basis to grow and become a stronger person.

Talents

We are each blessed with talents—the abilities that come naturally to an individual. Like many people, you may leave a talent lying in the background because you are not comfortable with it. To develop, though, you must learn to recognize all your talents and determine how they best benefit you. By using your talents, you strengthen them. For example, the major league baseball player strengthens his talents by hard work and practice. You need to do the same.

Knowledge

You are constantly learning and obtaining more knowledge. If you think you have stopped gaining knowledge, take time to re-evaluate your life. You absorb information daily—whether by observation, informal learning, or structured learning. The table on this page lists examples of each avenue of learning.

Self-directed learning is totally within your control. You can seek out tasks at work to expand your knowledge. Learning new tasks, functions, or positions at work is self-directed development.

Avenues of Learning

Observation   • Watching others complete tasks   • Watching others' reactions   • Watching mentors
Informal Learning   • Videos   • In-services   • Short presentations   • Self-directed learning
Structured Learning   • Classrooms   • Online classes   • Formal programs

Skills

Skills are learned and improve the more you use them. You can develop skills by a combination of using your talents and gaining knowledge. Put the components together and practice them, and your skill set will grow. Three of the most important skills you need to grow and succeed are these:

- Skill in communication
- Skill in writing
- Skill with people

One of the most important elements of using your skills is to make sure you are comfortable with them. The comfort only comes by practice and use. Do not be afraid to use your skills and make mistakes; that is how you learn and grow.

*You develop **skills** by using your **talents** and gaining **knowledge**.*

Advancement

According to Beverly Kaye and Sharon Jordan-Evans in their book *First, Break All the Rules,* you can make five possible moves *in addition* to moving up:

- ***Lateral Movement:*** Moving across or horizontally
- ***Re-alignment:*** Moving downward to open new opportunities
- ***Exploration:*** Temporary moves intended for researching other options
- ***Enrichment:*** Growing in place
- ***Re-location:*** Moving to another organization

Lateral movement occurs when you accept a position similar to your current one with little or no increased pay or benefits. Re-alignment is a method of moving down for a period of time so new opportunities are opened to you. If you have the opportunity to accept a temporary move in a new area, exploring it will help you decide if the new field is desirable to you. By assuming new responsibilities in your current position, you are growing in place. Deciding to leave your current organization is considered re-location.

To develop, you must be open to all possibilities when they are presented to you; as well, you must sometimes create your own options. Never be afraid of presenting a new option to your superiors after you have carefully researched the option.

Advancement often comes hand in hand with further formal education. Take a look at your options for pursuing a degree, certification, or apprenticeship (internship). Each of these avenues provides you with the opportunity to grow and progress.

Degree Programs

Degree programs are offered in many formats and many schedules. You can attend part-time, full-time, or one class at a time. You can take classes at an educational facility, online, or by videoconferencing. If you thought you could not make a schedule work to pursue higher education, explore that option again now. Never before have you had so many options to obtain a degree.

Certification Programs

Certification programs are offered by many different organizations. Look for certifications that are relevant to your profession and job-related activities. Research the certification and make sure it will benefit you. Some organizations that offer certifications are listed here along with their Internet addresses:

- International Association for Healthcare Security and Safety: www.iahss.org
- ASIS International: www.asis.org
- ECRI Institute: www.ecri.org
- American Society for Healthcare Engineering: www.ashe.org/ashe/about/mission/index.html
- Federal Emergency Management Agency: www.fema.gov

The IAHSS Web site notes that keeping current with standards and changes in the industry is important in protecting yourself against legal liability. Thus, you should generally renew your professional certifications or become certified at the next level every three to five years.

IAHSS Certification. This author would be remiss to omit describing the opportunities available through the IAHSS. If you are just starting out, look at the progressive certification program. This program takes you through several levels of certifications. You become certified by passing the exam for that level:

- Basic officer training
- Advanced officer training
- Supervisor training

Through the IAHSS, you can go on to obtain two additional levels of certification. For these, you must be or must have been the security, safety, or risk management administrator or manager of a healthcare facility; also, you must have earned the appropriate number of credits among the four categories of education, experience, membership, and specialized training. See the IAHSS Web site for details. These certifications are also earned in progression:

- Certified Healthcare Protection Administrator (CHPA)
- Certified Healthcare Protection Administrator-Fellow (CHPA-F)

Apprenticeships and Internships

Apprenticeship programs and internships are offered by states, local businesses, and hospitals. See what is available in your area and if it pertains to you. Often, community colleges grant credits toward your degree if you complete the formal apprenticeship program. Apprenticeship programs combine formal training with life knowledge and on-the-job experience.

Conclusion

You can accomplish whatever you choose to pursue. The key is to set your goals and pursue them. Remember, the options are plentiful; the only thing holding you back is yourself. Take the next step, and move forward in your personal and professional development. Pursue your dreams; the opportunities and ways to achieve them are at your finger tips.

Bibliography

Buckingham, M. and C. Coffman. 1999. *First, Break All the Rules.* New York: Simon & Schuster.

Buckingham, M. and D. O. Clifton. 2001. *Now, Discover Your Strengths.* New York: The Free Press.

International Association for Healthcare Security and Safety. IAHSS Certification—Renewal Process. On the Internet: www.iahss.org/cert_renewal.asp. Accessed 12 Jun 2007.

Kaye, B. and S. Jordan-Evans. 1999. *Love 'Em or Lose 'Em—Getting Good People To Stay.* San Francisco: Berrett-Koehler Publishers.

Study and Review Questions

1. Which of the following completes this statement? If you help others to grow in their profession, …

    A. …you will grow with them

    B. …you will be passed in their growth

    C. …you will not learn from it

    D. …you will not grow from it

2. Which of the following is not one of the three revolutionary tools needed to build a strong life?

    A. Understanding how to distinguish your natural talents

    B. A system to identify your dominant talents

    C. A common language to describe your talents

    D. An understanding of your options

3. Which of the following is not an example of structured learning?

    A. Classroom

    B. Online class

    C. Watching a mentor

    D. A formal program

4. In terms of advancement, how many possible moves are there in addition to moving up?

    A. Four

    B. Five

    C. Three

    D. Six

5. What does CHPA stand for?

    A. Certified Healthcare Professional Administrator

    B. Certified Hospital Protection Administrator

    C. Certified Healthcare Protection Administrator

    D. Certified Hospital Professional Administrator

IAHSS Progressive Certification Program

The Progressive Certification program of the IAHSS allows healthcare security personnel to continue their education after becoming certified at the Basic Training level. The Advanced and Supervisor Training levels expand on the Basic Training program. The following certifications are available:

- Basic Training certification for the healthcare security officer
- Advanced Training certification for the healthcare security officer
- Supervisor Training certification for the healthcare security professional

Each certification is valid for five years. Before the certification expires, the individual has the choice of being re-certified either by exam or through a point system.

Training Manuals

Information appropriate to certification for each level—Basic, Advanced, and Supervisor Training—is meticulously gathered in the IAHSS manual developed for that level:

- *Basic Training Manual for Healthcare Security Officers*
- *Advanced Training Manual*
- *Supervisor Training Manual for Healthcare Security Personnel*

Who Can Take the Exams?

All healthcare security officers and those aspiring to work in healthcare security and safety are eligible to start the certification process beginning with the Basic Training level. Successful completion of the Basic Training certification extends eligibility to progress to the Advanced Training level and then to the Supervisor Training level

Online Exams

Online Exams are available for purchase at: http://iahss.proexams.com

IAHSS Supervisor Training Manual for Healthcare Security Personnel

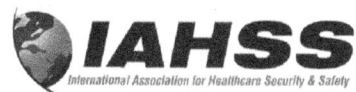

Application for Written Examination

Supervisor Training Certification Examination, Third Edition

To order a written examination, complete the Applicant Information/Senior Member Information and remit with the fee of $80.00.

Office Use Only
Date Received _____ Date Sent _____
Senior Member Status Verified By_____
Examination Serial Number_____

Please use this address if mailing your application and payment:

IAHSS
PO Box 5038
Glendale Heights IL 60139
888/353-0990 • 630/529-3913 • Fax 630/529-4139

Note: The examination paper is only valid for 45 days from the date of issue.
THIS APPLICATION MAY BE REPRODUCED

Applicant Information (print clearly):

Social Security Number_____

Name (first and last)_____

Mailing address_____

City State ZIP_____

Telephone_____

E-mail_____

Senior Member Information (print clearly):

Name (first and last)_____

Mailing Address_____

City State ZIP_____

Telephone_____ Fax_____

E-mail_____

I request the paper examination for the award of certification for the IAHSS Supervisor Training program. I have contacted the Senior Member above, who has agreed to administer this time-limited, closed-book examination to me. I understand I must answer at least 70% of the questions correctly to be certified for a five-year period. The fee of $80.00 (US funds) is enclosed with this completed application form.
I understand there is no refund of this fee should I fail to obtain a passing score to be certified and that a new application form and fee must be submitted for re-examination.

Applicant Signature_____
                                                                                            Date

Senior Member Signature_____
                                                                                            Date